TUTI TEN
AND THE JOURNEY
OF HOPE

Threads of Resilience

CYNETHEA CUNNINGHAM

TUTI TENDER-HEART AND THE JOURNEY OF HOPE

© 2024 by CYNETHEA CUNNINGHAM

Dove Inspired Publications
Rockville, Maryland
For information, please e-mail
roundaboutwednesday@gmail.com

Printed in the United States
First Printing Edition, 2024

DEDICATION

In Loving Memory of
Mildred Hazel Walker
June 6, 1948 to September 12, 1987

Thank you for your support and encouragement. May this story of Tuti and Tia inspire you with hope and resilience. And remember if a cloth doll can handle life's challenges, so can we! 😊

"With Warmest Regards"

CONTENTS

*Resilience in Adversity is
the Essence of Hope*

INTRODUCTION

Millie sat beside Tia on the edge of her bed, her soft voice filled with love. Tia's eyes widened as she looked at her mother, who bore the weight of a thousand unspoken words.

"What is it, Momma?" Tia asked softly.

"I have breast cancer," Millie said. "The doctors tried everything but couldn't stop it, and now it's too late for a cure."

Tia's lower lip quivered. "Are you going away, Momma?"

Millie's gaze softened. "Oh, my precious Tia," she said softly, with tenderness and sorrow in her eyes. "I wish I could stay, but Heaven calls for me."

Millie reached for the brown cloth doll sitting on the nearby chair—a creation of love and hope. "This," Millie said, "is Tuti Tender-Heart. Tuti is a special doll that will offer you comfort and companionship. You can hold her close when I'm gone and know my love remains with you."

As the days turned into weeks, Millie's strength waned. Tia clung to Tuti Tender-Heart, finding comfort in its worn embrace. And when Millie took her last breath, Tia felt the legacy pass—a torch of love from mother to daughter.

Tia held Tuti close, knowing she would soon face a world without Millie. Its stitches may fray, but the comfort remains. And in the quiet moments when grief threatens to overwhelm her, Tia feels her mother's presence—the echo of a love that surpasses time.

Dear reader, let us step into their story—a tale of courage, legacy, and the enduring bond between a mother, her daughter, and a cherished cloth doll named Tuti Tender-Heart. It's a journey that inspires both past and present, woven into a rich fabric of love and hope.

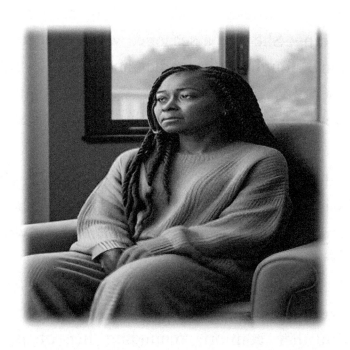

Contemplating the emotional landscape of a mother confronting her mortality and the legacy she hopes to leave behind.

Chapter One: A Storm Within

Millie sat by the window, tracing raindrops as they raced down the glass pane. Outside, the world blurred—a soft gray like a watercolor painting. But within her chest, a storm brewed, fierce and unyielding. She was a seasoned warrior, accustomed to battles fought with needles and threads, stitching together lives and stories. Yet this battle was different—a relentless storm threatening to consume her.

The doctor delivered the diagnosis with clinical precision, leaving little room for hope. The cure, elusive as a distant shore, taunted her. Millie wore her determination like armor, trying to stay strong for Tia. But beneath the surface, a storm of fear, anger, and resolve raged within her. The scent of lavender brought her comfort, reminding her of peaceful evenings and sunny fields. Despite the turmoil, that fragrance anchored her, a sign that tough times would pass. Her tea sat forgotten on the side table, its chamomile aroma a bittersweet presence. Rain streaked the window, blurring the outside world, leaving Millie to wonder if hope could shine through.

Caught between raindrops and memories, Millie sat waiting for her inner turmoil to settle. Her fingers sought solace on the cool, smooth glass of the window frame. The rain's gentle patter was soothing, and Tia's laughter echoed in her mind, a fragile melody that both comforted and saddened her. It reminded her of moments slipping away, like raindrops on a windowpane. How could she leave behind this precious child, this extension of her heart?

Her gaze lingered on the family photos lining the windowsill—their smiles preserved in frames, memories etched in pixels. Millie longed to freeze time, to hold those moments close. The mingling scent of lavender and old books brought her back to the present. Each tick of the clock, unyielding and unsympathetic, stole fragments of her life, its steady and unchanging beat a painful reminder of the passing of time.

Persistent fear settled in Millie's mind, a haunting ache that clung to her thoughts. The idea of leaving Tia weighed heavily, casting a shadow over graduations, wedding days, and all the pivotal moments she would miss. Millie dreaded the absence of shared laughter and hushed conversations—the intimate threads that bound them. But above all, she feared becoming just a distant memory in her daughter's heart.

In quiet moments, Millie envisioned her voice resonating in Tia's laughter, her touch lingering in every hug, and the sparkle in Tia's eyes as they shared dreams and secrets. She yearned to witness Tia's milestones, to stand by her through challenges and victories, and to cheer from the sidelines, steadfast in her support no matter the path Tia chose. The ache in her heart intensified, knowing that time was slipping away like sand through her fingers.

Despite everything, Millie clung to memories: late nights lying side by side gazing at the glow-in-the-dark stars on Tia's bedroom ceiling; the scent of Tia's hair after a bath; the warmth of her small hands in hers; the sound of her giggles as they danced around the living room; and the way she softly said, "I love you, Momma," before drifting off to sleep. These fragments of their shared experience were her lifeline—tethers to a life slipping away.

Amid her turmoil, Millie clung to hope as a fragile lifeline to Tia's future. She vowed to leave behind notes and photographs, capturing their moments of joy. Millie wanted Tia to always feel her love, no matter where life took them. As Tia approached the threshold of her own journey, Millie wished with all her heart that her daughter would sense the enduring presence of love guiding her forward.

Regret washed over Millie as she reflected on the ignored warning signs: the dismissed lump, the fatigue attributed to stress. Now those signs echoed loudly. She wished she had listened to the subtle hints from her body and sought help sooner.

Grief draped around Millie like a fragile shawl, woven from threads of unexperienced moments she would never live. The art classes remained mere sketches in her mind, Hawaiian sunsets forever out of reach, and the cobblestone streets of Paris—places she'd only wander through in her dreams. In the quietness of night, her silent tears soaked the soft pillow.

Even in her moments of grief, Millie clung to hope. She believed Tia would find peace, knowing her momma was in a better place. Millie understood that a mother's love transcends time. Their bond, formed through both joy and sorrow, became a cherished collection of memories. She prayed these memories would guide Tia through life's challenges.

Hope spoke to Millie, weaving delicate threads of longing. She prayed Tia would cherish the echo of her laughter, the comforting warmth of her presence, and the gospel songs hummed while stirring pots in the kitchen. In a poignant moment, as the pot bubbled and the rich aroma of spices filled the air, Tia's curious eyes widened. "Momma," she asked, her voice filled with wonder, "why does your gumbo taste like a hug?" Millie would wink, her heart swelling, and reply, "Because, my sweet girl, it's seasoned with love." This bittersweet yet cherished memory seasoned their days with joy.

Millie hoped Tia would remember the warmth of their home, the scent of freshly baked bread, and the gentle touch of her hands. She wished Tia would recall how her voice filled the house with love and the moments they shared. Each memory was a thread in their lives, weaving an unbreakable bond between mother and daughter.

Under the weight of mortality, Millie wrote a heartfelt letter—a promise in ink. She shared her hopes, dreams, and life lessons, each word filled with cherished memories, laughter, and love. In her delicate script, she recounted times she rose above challenges with grace. Millie's letter was more than just words; it was a reflection of her life for Tia. She spoke of finding beauty in small moments, the power of kindness, and holding onto love even in tough times. Her letter became a timeless legacy, a source of comfort and inspiration, reminding Tia that her spirit would always be with her, guiding her through life's challenges with love:

My Dearest Tia,

As I sit here, pen in hand, I think of you—the way your eyes light up when you discover something new, the warmth of your hand in mine. You are my greatest joy, my heart's song. Life, my dear daughter, is like a patchwork quilt, with love-stitched memories filling each square. In this letter, I put those memories into words.

Remember the day we danced in the rain? Your laughter echoed through the puddles, and I realized that happiness is a simple thing—a splash of water, a shared secret, a hug that lingers. Life isn't always easy, my love. There will be storms, but you are stronger than you know. When the winds howl, find shelter in kindness. It's a soft blanket that warms the soul. I have faced many challenges, and each time, I found strength in love and grace. Hold onto love, even in the darkest times for it will guide you through.

Tia, your dreams are like stars in the night sky. Reach for them. Imagine far-off lands and adventures carried by the wind. Dream until your heart overflows with possibility. Remember this: You are loved beyond measure. Your heart, a treasure chest of courage and wonder, holds the keys to countless doors. Open them fearlessly.

With all my heart,

Momma

Millie poured her heart into the letter, creating a legacy of love for Tia. With a tender smile, she sealed the envelope with a kiss and placed it in a special handcrafted wooden box. This box passed down from her mother, had once stored family heirlooms and precious memories. Now, Millie filled it with keepsakes for Tia—a locket with their pictures, a dried rose from their garden, and a hand-stitched quilt.

The patterns of blooming flowers and twinkling stars symbolized the beauty and hope Millie wished to impart. Each item was a piece of their shared history, a tangible reminder of their bond. As she closed the box, Millie said a silent prayer, hoping her daughter would always feel her love and guidance, even in her absence.

As rain tapped the window, she softly prayed, "Dear Lord, watch over my dear girl. May she feel Your comforting presence and my love." In the serene room, love and sorrow came together, crafting a masterpiece in a mother's heart.

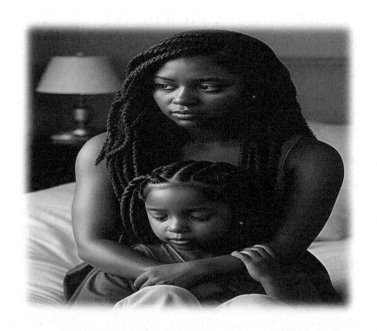

Reflecting on the timeless bond between
a mother and her child.

Chapter Two: Millie's Eternal Promise

The rain had ceased, and the sun emerged from behind the clouds. Millie sat beside Tia on the edge of her bed, her voice gentle and loving. Sunlight danced through the room, caressing the quilted fabric that adorned her bed—a quilt lovingly crafted by Tia's grandmother. Precious moments wove a mosaic of generations within that quilt, creating a cherished legacy.

Tia's eyes widened as she looked at her mother. Millie's face carried the weight of a thousand unspoken words. Brushing a strand of hair from Tia's forehead, she said, "Oh, my sweet girl," her voice trembling, "Sometimes life throws storms our way. But we're warriors, you and me. We fight, even when the world feels heavy."

Tia nodded, her heart fluttering. She sensed something was wrong—her mother's wavering smile and the hesitant breaths she took when she thought no one was looking. "Momma," Tia asked softly, "Why are you sad?"

Millie's eyes softened, and she reached for Tia's hand. Her gaze shifted to the cherished Bible resting on the nightstand. "You know how sometimes people get sick, right?"

Tia vividly recalled Grandma's battle with the flu the previous year. Her voice remained steady, yet emotions swirled beneath the surface. "Yes," she replied. "But sometimes, the sickness can be far more serious." Millie hesitated, then said the words that weighed heavily on her heart: "I have breast cancer."

The words hung in the air, thick and unmoving. Tia's eyes widened as she absorbed the news. "Breast cancer?" she said, her voice trembling. "Is that like having a monster inside you?"

Millie tried to smile, despite the tears threatening to spill. "Not exactly, my love. It's like… like a storm. A storm that's been raging inside me."

Tears welled up in Tia's eyes. "But storms go away, right?" she asked, her voice full of hope.

Millie's heart clenched. "Sometimes, yes. But this storm… it's stronger than I thought. The doctors tried everything but couldn't stop it, and now it's too late for a cure."

Tia's lower lip quivered. "Are you going away, Momma?"

Millie's gaze softened, and she took a deep breath. "Oh, my precious Tia," she said gently. "I wish I could stay, but Heaven calls for me."

Tia's tears spilled out, and she clung to Millie's hand. "No," she choked out. "You can't leave me."

Millie pulled Tia into her arms, holding her tightly. "I'm not leaving just yet sweet girl. But soon, I'll have to go to a place where the pain stops. A place where I won't be sick anymore."

Tia buried her face in Millie's chest, her small frame trembling with sobs. "I don't want you to go, Momma," she said, her voice choked with emotion.

Millie's tears flowed freely, tracing silent paths down her cheeks. She cradled Tia's head against her shoulder, her touch gentle yet firm. "I know, baby." she said softly, "But listen carefully. Even when I'm not here, the Lord will watch over you. He'll be your guardian, your guiding light."

Tia's eyes, red and swollen, lifted to meet Millie's gaze. "The Lord?" she asked, tone tinged with doubt. Millie's voice was a soft breeze, barely audible. "Yes," she said. "When you're scared or worried, just talk to God. He'll be right there with you, just like Momma said. And at night, when you see the glimmering stars, know it's me sending you all my love."

Tia's eyes mirrored Millie's own. "Will you be with Him?" she asked, her voice a fragile thread of wonder and longing.

Millie nodded, her eyes fixed on the distant horizon. "Yes, my love. I'll always be with Him, watching over you."

Side by side, mother and daughter sat wrapped in a warm embrace of love and faith. Millie's fingers gently brushed against Tia's hair as she began softly singing a song—a melody passed down from her mother. The words spoke of a love that surpassed time.

In the quiet of night, when stars shine so bright,
They whisper secrets to the moon's soft light.
Ancient songs bring comfort, whispers of love,
Thru valleys and mountains, under the moon above.

Guided by unseen hands, love takes flight,
A flame that burns forever, oh so bright.
When storms rage and tears blur our sight,
These sacred notes guide us through the night.

Love dances in our hearts, wiping away fears,
It's a melody that lasts beyond earthly years.
So listen, my sweet Tia, to this song that echoes through time,
And know you are cradled in love that is truly sublime,
And in love's embrace, our spirits align.

Millie's soft voice faded into the night, leaving a melody that would forever echo in Tia's heart. The shadows enveloped the room, casting a gentle hush over their shared moment. Beyond the window, a solitary star twinkled—a promise kept, a testament to a mother's boundless love. As the night deepened, the star's light seemed to grow brighter, a beacon of hope and a reminder of the unbreakable bond between mother and daughter.

Millie's lullaby lingered in the air, wrapping Tia in warmth and comfort. As the soft melody drifted through the room, Tia nestled closer to her mother, feeling the gentle touch of her arms. In the quiet, Tia felt her mother's love and guidance, a light that would always stay with her. Their bond was unbreakable, a source of strength and love that would last a lifetime.

In that sacred space, love and sadness came together, creating something beautiful within a mother's heart. They lingered there—a daughter bound to memories, a mother passing down her legacy. The song of their bond echoed, fragile yet everlasting.

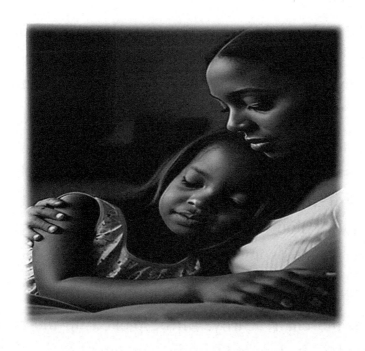

Embracing the tender bond between a mother, her child, and the warmth of love.

Chapter Three: An Enduring Bond

Tia gently rested her head on Millie's shoulder, inhaling the comforting scent of lavender. Her tears flowed as she said softly, "I don't want to lose you, Momma."

Millie embraced Tia, her voice gentle and comforting. "You won't lose me, Tia. My love will always be with you, even when I'm not here. It will wrap around you like a warm blanket."

Tia leaned up against her mother, her eyes wide with curiosity and a touch of sadness. The room, bathed in the soft glow of the nightlight, held an intimate warmth. "You know," she said softly, "you're not alone. There's someone else here to comfort you, too."

"Who, Momma?" she asked, wiping her tears.

From the chair nearby, Millie picked up the brown cloth doll. Its braided yarn hair matched Tia's, and its hand-drawn eyes shone with kindness. The stitched smile offered comfort.

Millie's voice was soft and tender as she spoke. "This is Tuti Tender-Heart, your special doll."

Tia held Tuti close, the fabric's softness brushing against her cheek.

"Why is Tuti so special?" she asked.

"Because," Millie said softly, "your Aunt Cynethea made Tuti with love. Tuti carries hope and comfort. Even in the toughest moments, there's always hope. Hold her close when I'm gone; she'll remind you of my love."

Tia's hand traced the delicate details on Tuti's fabric features: the bright eyes, the stitched smile, and the delicate pink heart on her chest.

She quietly said, "Thank you, Momma."

Millie's smile grew tender as her fingers brushed against Tia's hair. "When fear or loneliness tiptoe in," she said softly, "speak to Tuti. She'll listen, just like I do."

She gently kissed Tia's forehead. "Remember, my brave girl, the Lord will watch over you from Heaven, and Tuti will be at your side."

Tia's eyes welled up with tears, her heart aching at the thought of losing her momma. She clutched the Tuti Tender-Heart doll tightly, seeking comfort in its presence.

"I'll miss you so much, Momma," she said, trembling.

"I'll miss you too, my precious daughter."

As days stretched into weeks, Millie's strength waned in her fierce battle against breast cancer. Tia clung to hope, her heart aching as she witnessed her mother's struggle—each hard breath a painful reminder. Yet, deep down, she sensed her mother slipping away, like a fragile whisper carried by the wind. In the hospital room, weeks blurred into days as Millie's strength continued to fade. Tia held her mother's hand during each draining chemotherapy session. The rhythmic beeping of the IV pump punctuated the silence—a soundtrack of uncertainty.

Tia imagined chemotherapy as a potent elixir coursing through Millie's veins, battling cancer cell by cell. By her bedside, she offered a silent prayer. But reality remained unyielding: Millie's once-lustrous hair was now a memory, and her labored breaths revealed life's delicate balance between fighting and surrendering.

Tia, wise beyond her years, knew the truth: despite the hospital visits, treatments, and fervent wishes, her mother was slipping away. Cancer stole moments, memories, and dreams. Yet, in quiet hand-holding moments, Tia felt a bond—a fragile flame flickering in the darkness. In that peaceful room, as the inevitable unfolded, Millie closed her eyes, enveloped by love and the whisper of eternity, and took her final breath.

Tia clutched Tuti tightly, her tears saturating the doll's fabric. Despite her sorrow, she sensed her momma's touch—a bond that would last long after Millie was gone.

As days turned into weeks, Tuti remained steadfast by Tia's side. Each morning, Tia would wake to find Tuti nestled against her pillow, her sad face absorbing the remnants of grief that clung to the room. The stitched-on expression seemed to echo Tia's heartache, a silent witness to her pain.

But Tuti also had another face—a happy one. When sorrow weighed heavily on Tia, she would turn Tuti around, revealing the smiling countenance. It was as if the doll brought hope into the quiet corner of the room. Even in darkness, there was a light to be found—a glimmer of possibility, a promise that joy could still bloom. Tuti became Tia's constant companion. She sat in the same chair by the window, just as Momma used to do. Through changing seasons, Tia found solace in the doll's presence. Love, she realized, goes beyond the boundaries of life and death. Her momma's spirit endured within the delicate stitches of Tuti's fabric—a comforting connection bridging past and present.

Outside the window, the world continued its dance. Leaves turned crimson, then surrendered to the earth. Snowflakes dusted the windowpane, and spring buds gently opened, revealing delicate petals.

Tia observed it all, her fingers tracing the familiar patterns on Tuti's face. She wondered if Momma saw these same seasons from where she was.

One night, as the moon hung low, and the stars blinked like distant lanterns, Tia softly asked, "Momma, are you there? Can you hear me?"

As Tia gazed out her window, a shooting star streaked across the night sky. Her breath caught, recognizing it as Momma's promise—a celestial gift of hope and guidance, briefly illuminating the darkness.

Tia's heart swelled with the memory of Momma's promise that her love would wrap around her like a warm blanket. She could feel the warmth of that love.

In her room, love and sorrow blended, creating something profound within Tia's heart. She closed her eyes, cocooned in the timeless embrace of their enduring bond.

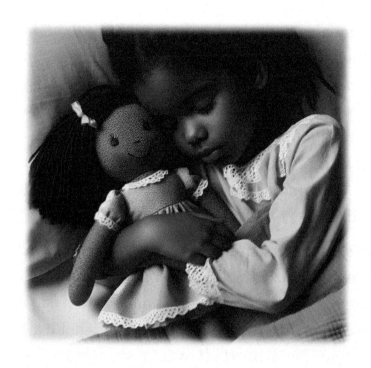

*Finding comfort in the soothing bonds
of unexpected companionship.*

Chapter Four: A Comforting Companion

After Millie passed away, sorrow filled Tia's life. Breast cancer claimed her mother, leaving behind an overwhelming ache. Each morning, she woke to the quiet emptiness of the house—the absence of Momma's laughter, the lingering scent of lavender (Momma's favorite), and the memory of breakfast aromas that once filled the kitchen. Tia missed her Momma's voice calling from the bottom of the stairs saying, "Good morning, Sweet Tia, it's time to rise and shine!" Pushing back her cozy covers, she would say, "Yes, ma'am," and shuffle to the window to greet the day.

Tia's room became a sanctuary of memories. The walls adorned with photographs captured her mother's tender smile—a portal to the past. Among these cherished images, one picture held a special place in Tia's heart. It was a snapshot of her and Momma in the garden, both laughing as they planted lavender together. Momma's eyes sparkled with joy and Tia's face was lit up with pure happiness. This treasured photo in a delicate lavender-colored frame, sat on Tia's bedside table, a cherished memory of their shared moments.

The quilt on her bed was a cherished family heirloom, lovingly handmade by Tia's grandmother and given to Millie as a wedding gift. Each patch told a story, stitched together from pieces of old dresses, baby blankets, and even some of Momma's favorite aprons. The quilt was a tangible piece of Momma's love, keeping Tia warm on countless nights. Its worn, soft fabric was a testament to the many years of comfort it had provided.

The subtle scent of Momma's perfume clung to the folds of the worn quilt, enveloping Tia in a comforting embrace. Momma's perfume was a delicate blend of lavender and vanilla, a scent that was both soothing and warm. It always made Tia feel safe and happy. Whenever Tia caught a whiff of that familiar scent, it was as if Momma was right there beside her.

Despite the ache, Tia found small comforts in her memories. She would wrap herself in Momma's old quilt, feeling a semblance of her embrace. The scent of lavender, though faint, brought a sense of closeness to Momma. Every night, as she lay in bed, Tia would whisper, "Goodnight, Momma," hoping that somehow, Momma could hear her. These small, yet profoundly meaningful connections helped Tia navigate the difficult days and keep her mother's memory alive.

The days felt long and heavy without Momma. Tia often found herself wandering through the house, touching the things Momma had loved. The old rocking chair by the window, where Momma used to sit and read, now stood silent. The scent of lavender still lingered faintly in the air, mingling with the smell of old books and polished wood. The soft creak of the floorboards under her feet and the distant chirping of birds outside the window added to the stillness. Tia could almost hear the rustle of pages as Momma turned them, and the gentle sound of her voice reading aloud. The warmth of the quilt, the coolness of the polished wood, and the faint taste of salt from her tears all combined to create a vivid tapestry of memories.

However, it was Tuti Tender-Heart that occupied the most profound corner of Tia's heart—a cherished gift of love and connection, a tangible reminder of her mother's presence even in her absence. Tuti was more than just a doll; she was a confidante, a source of comfort, and a symbol of the unbreakable bond between Tia and her Momma. Every time Tia held Tuti, she felt a sense of closeness to her mother, as if Momma's love was stitched into every seam. Tuti's presence provided comfort on the loneliest nights and strength during the hardest days, showing the lasting love that went beyond even the greatest loss.

Under the soft moonlight, Tia lay in bed, thinking about Momma. She missed their secrets, bedtime stories, and tales of Momma's childhood. Most of all, she missed the warm hugs at night. Tia reached for the doll, touching its soft fabric. In that quiet moment, seeking comfort, she said, "I miss Momma so much." Tears filled her eyes, ready to fall. Tuti's sad face seemed to understand. Softly, Tia asked, "Why, Tuti, did Momma have to go?" Tuti's kind eyes seemed to know all about sadness and missing someone.

To her amazement, Tuti leaned towards her, and in a gentle voice, she replied, "Your Momma loved you more than anything, Tia. She's still here, watching over you."

Tia's eyes widened. "Tuti, you can talk?"

Tuti smiled. "Yes, Tia. I've always been here to listen, but now you need more than that. I'm here to help you remember your Momma's love and remind you that you are never alone."

"I was made with love and purpose," Tuti explained. "When you hold me, I'm more than just fabric. I carry your feelings, whether you're sad or happy."

Tia's eyes filled with tears as she listened. "When you miss your Momma, I hold that feeling for you. And when you cry, I feel your tears." Tia blinked, touched by the doll's words. She felt a warmth spreading through her chest—a small comfort in her grief. "Thank you, Tuti. You make me feel like Momma is still here with me."

Tuti nodded. "She is, Tia. Her love is always with you, in your heart and your memories."

Tia looked at Tuti with a mix of wonder and gratitude. "How can I keep going without Momma?"

Tuti's eyes softened. "By remembering her love and letting it guide you. She would want you to be happy and to live your life fully. And whenever you need a reminder, I'll be here."

Tuti's eyes twinkled, her voice soft and comforting: "Remember her laughter, her warmth. Carry her spirit with you. And when the nights are darkest, I'll be here—a reminder of her love. My purpose is to help you find comfort and to be a bridge between your heart and your Momma's love. Whenever you feel lost or alone, just hold me close, and know that Momma's love is always with you. Together, we'll get through this, my dear Tia."

As the nights went by, Tuti became a constant presence in Tia's life. They talked about Momma's strength, her laughter, and the gospel songs she loved. Tia listened closely, and her heart slowly began to heal. Love connected them, linking the past and present. Tia held onto Tuti, finding comfort in the memories. The pain was still there but knowing that love never fades made it easier.

Days turned into weeks, and as the seasons changed, Tia found comfort in Tuti's presence. She found small ways to honor her mother's memory. Together, they planted lavender in the garden, filling the air with its soothing scent. Each bloom was a tribute to Momma, a reminder of their shared love and the beautiful moments they had spent together.

One sunny afternoon, while tending to the lavender plants, Tia noticed a butterfly fluttering around her. It landed gently on her hand. She remembered Momma saying that butterflies were messengers of love and hope. Tia smiled and softly said, "Thank you, Momma." When the wind rustled the leaves, Tia imagined it carried Momma's soft voice, gently saying, "You're never alone, my sweet Tia."

In her quiet room, Tia held Tuti and realized she didn't have to carry her grief alone. A calmness settled within her, knowing that love stays even after someone is gone. Memories, like delicate flowers, showed the special bond between a mother and her daughter.

Even though Tia still felt the ache of loss, she found comfort in small moments of connection. Tuti Tender-Heart became a source of strength and love. Tia knew that Momma's spirit would always guide her through the days ahead.

With her eyes gently shut, bathed in silvery moonlight, Tia felt her momma's continuous presence. The room echoed with laughter, bedtime stories, and shared secrets. And as the moon traced its arc across the sky, Tia said softly, "I love you, Momma, always."

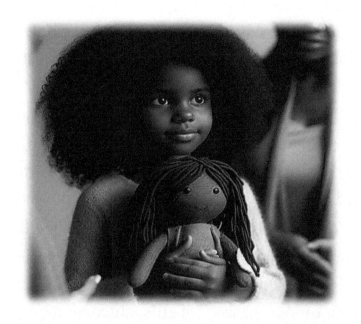

Drawing inspiration from those who transform pain into purpose, and the quiet advocates who raise their voices for a cause.

Chapter Five: Echoes Of Hope

Even though breast cancer took her mother too soon and forever changed her world, hope blossomed within Tia. Amidst the sorrow, a comforting presence emerged: Tuti Tender-Heart. Lovingly crafted by Tia's aunt, every stitch in the doll was a tribute to her momma's warmth, humor, and courage during her battle against breast cancer.

Tia could sense her mother's spirit woven into the doll's fabric as she cradled it close. The setting sun cast a warm glow on her mother's well-worn scarf draped around her shoulders. Tuti lay on a nearby pillow, her bright eyes reflecting understanding.

In a hushed voice, Tia said, "Momma used to say that love is like sunshine—it warms even the coldest corners of our hearts." Tuti's stitched mouth was curved in a smile. "Your Momma was wise, my dear. She left behind more than memories—she left you with a purpose."

Tia furrowed her brow, lost in thought.

"A purpose? What purpose could that be?"

Tuti's eyes sparkled. "To raise awareness," Tuti said, "so other families don't have to endure the same pain."

As Tia listened to Tuti's words, a mix of thoughts and emotions filled her. She felt a bit unsure but also curious, wondering how she could help others despite her young age.

"But how?" Tia asked. "I'm just a child."

Tia's mind was full of thoughts. She remembered watching her Momma cheer others up while bravely fighting breast cancer. Momma's strength and kindness had helped so many people, and Tia wondered if she could ever be as brave and strong as her.

"But what if I'm not strong enough? Tia said, her voice trembling.

Tuti leaned closer. "Tia," she said gently, "you are very wise for your age. You carry your mother's strength and kindness. One day, you will stand tall and use your voice to help others learn about breast cancer and bring hope."

Tia pulled her momma's scarf snugly around her, seeking comfort in its familiar embrace. The lingering scent of lavender and memories enveloped her, and she said softly, "But it hurts, Tuti. How can I do this without her?"

Tuti placed a comforting hand on Tia's shoulder. "Your momma lives on in you. Every time you share her story, every time you encourage someone to get screened, she's there," Tia closed her eyes, imagining her momma's gentle, soothing voice. "Tia, my love, life is like a quilt. Each stitch matters, no matter how small."

Gently placing her hand on Tia's chest, Tuti said, "Strength comes from the heart, Tia. You have a heart full of love and courage. Every small step you take, every kind word you share, will make a difference. You don't have to do it all at once. Just be yourself and let your love for Momma guide you. She's always with you, guiding you with her love."

Tia felt a warm feeling in her heart. She realized that even though she was a child, she could still carry on Momma's love in her special way. She could start by telling her story, planting more lavender, and being kind and caring to everyone around her.

As she thought about these things, she felt a mix of emotions. She felt proud and happy, knowing she could make a difference. Sometimes, she felt a little sad, missing her momma. But this sadness was mixed with a comforting feeling like her momma's love was always with her. Tia imagined the beautiful lavender plants growing, each one a symbol of her momma's love and strength. She saw herself sharing her momma's story with friends and new people, spreading hope and kindness. Tia knew that her small acts of kindness could create ripples of love and support and touch many lives. This made her feel determined and glad, knowing she could especially honor her momma's memory.

Tia was confident that, with Tuti at her side, she would one day discover her voice and make a meaningful difference, just like her Momma. And in that moment, she felt a little less alone, knowing that Momma's spirit was always with her, guiding her throughout her journey.

Tia looked at Tuti, her voice soft. "Momma used to say that everything in life has a purpose—even you, dear Tuti."

That night, Tia made a special promise. "I will honor Momma's memory, not with tears, but with a purpose," she said softly. "I will speak up and help others learn about breast cancer. Every step I take and every word I speak will show Momma's strength.

Tuti quietly nodded, her heart filled with love. Tia felt warm inside imagining herself talking to friends, sharing stories about her momma, and helping people understand how to support those with breast cancer. She pictured the smiles on their faces as they listened, the way their eyes would light up with understanding and compassion. Tia knew that by sharing her momma's journey she could make a difference, spreading awareness and kindness wherever she went.

The next morning, Tia woke up with a sense of determination. She started by planting a small garden of lavender, just like Momma loved. As she carefully placed each seed in the soil, she whispered, "This is for you, Momma." Tuti watched from her cozy spot, her heart glowing brighter with each seed Tia planted.

Under the same moon that had seen her cry, Tia promised to be strong. She would honor her momma, herself, and everyone fighting against breast cancer. With Tuti by her side, Tia knew she could make a difference, one small step at a time.

And so, Tia's journey began, filled with hope, love, and the strength of her momma's memory. Every day, she took a step closer to her promise, touching hearts and inspiring others, just like her momma did.

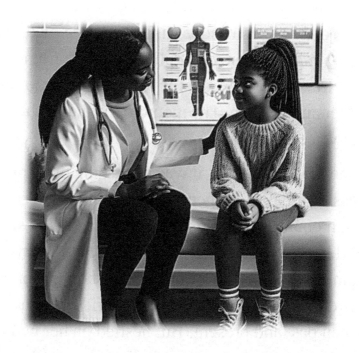

Dedicated to all the brave souls who educate themselves, advocate for awareness, and carry the torch.

Chapter Six: A Quest For Truth

Tia's room remained unchanged—a cozy cocoon of memories. The patchwork quilt her grandmother had stitched adorned the bed, while faded posters of constellations and fairy tales held secrets from her childhood. Once proudly displayed, the pictures of her momma now rested in delicate picture frames. Tia would trace their edges as if touching her momma's laughter and warmth. The memories clung to the walls like ivy seeking solace.

Ah, the wooden floor—it was more than mere planks. It was a lullaby, a gentle hum that cradled Tia through countless nights. Its creaks held secrets shared only with those who listened closely. Tia imagined her momma's footsteps echoing alongside hers, dancing across the floor, bridging the gap between past and present. But nestled on her bed, was the most treasured secret of all: Tuti, her cloth doll—a heartfelt gift from her mother, that brought comfort during countless tearful moments.

Tia sat in the chair by the window, sunlight peeking through the curtains. She held Tuti gently, her fingers tracing the stitches that kept Tuti's heart safe. And in that quiet moment, Tia wondered whether love could be stitched too. Her momma's laughter echoed in the room, a bittersweet melody that danced with the dust motes.

Bathed in the warm embrace of sunlight, Tia remained seated in her chair, her eyes fixed on the window, while her thoughts roamed far beyond the glass pane. The world beyond beckoned—a realm of uncertainties and revelations. She was no longer the little girl who believed in magic and happy ever after. The whispers of adulthood had grown louder, and they carried weight.

Her momma's absence felt like a shadow. The cancer had taken her away, leaving behind a space in the house. Tia's fingers gently stroked Tuti's hair, wondering if she would face the same thing. Would this disease take her too?

The adults had tiptoed around the truth, their voices hushed, their answers evasive. Tia yearned for clarity—the facts that could pierce through the fog of uncertainty. She needed to understand, to confront the monster that had claimed her mother. Today, she resolved to change things. No more whispers; she would seek clear answers. With determination and a thirst for knowledge, she stepped out of her room and into the world, ready to uncover what she needed to know.

The local clinic stood nestled between the bakery and the flower shop, its aged yet inviting sign swaying gently in the breeze. As Tia pushed open the door, the bell chimed, announcing her arrival. In the waiting area, patients peacefully gazed at magazines while awaiting their turn. Some chatted softly with each other, sharing stories and laughter. A few children played with toys in a corner, their giggles filling the room. A woman with a gentle smile knitted a colorful scarf, her needles moving swiftly and steadily. The atmosphere was calm and comforting, a small haven of warmth and care.

Dr. Sherece emerged from her office, kind eyes framed by a stethoscope draped around her neck. Tia felt a sense of comfort as she extended her hand and greeted her. "Tia," Dr. Sherece said, "welcome. How can I assist you today?" Tia's voice wavered. "I want to know about breast cancer. What are the signs? How can I protect myself?"

Dr. Sherece led her into an examination room with detailed anatomical diagrams on the walls. As they sat together on the long padded bench, Dr. Sherece began, "Tia, cancer is like a rogue artist. It creates chaos within our bodies. Cells multiply uncontrollably, forming tumors. But we fight back with chemotherapy, radiation, and surgery. Sometimes we win; sometimes we lose. Our canvas is hope, and our brushstrokes are resilience."

Tia listened intently, her heart beating like a drum. She absorbed information about breast cancer stages, survival rates, and the indomitable strength of the human spirit. Dr. Sherece spoke of hope, research breakthroughs, and the occasional setbacks faced in this battle. Tia's questions flowed freely, like a river seeking its course.

"And what about me?" Tia finally asked. "Will cancer take me too?"

Dr. Sherece's gaze softened. "We can't predict the future, Tia. But knowledge is your armor. Learn, ask, and live. Your mother lives on within you—in your courage."

Dr. Sherece thoroughly educated Tia about breast self-examination, emphasizing the significance of understanding her own body. Tia resolved to incorporate a monthly breast self-examination routine into her life, dedicating 15 minutes to this crucial practice.

Tia's heart raced as she absorbed the information. Leaving the clinic with pamphlets in hand, she felt empowered by this newfound understanding. She resolved to confront fear with knowledge and, in her mother's honor, vowed never to remain silent. As she returned home, the sun bathed her face, and the weight of responsibility settled upon her.

In her cozy bedroom, Tia stood by the window, her gaze fixed on ever-shifting clouds pirouetting across the sky. With a soft, determined voice, she said, "I won't yield to fear, Momma. I'll learn, I'll fight, and I'll live." Earnest resolve, inner strength, and a deep desire to honor her mother ignited Tia's determination. The ache of loss and a promise she made to herself, became the gentle breeze lifting her spirit. In that quiet moment by the window, as clouds danced gracefully across the sky, Tia discovered a hidden strength that blossomed with hope.

In that room where childhood met adulthood, Tia's coming-of-age journey began—a search for answers, a battle against shadows, and a symphony of courage. Her quest was driven by love, filled with hope, and guided by the comforting words of Dr. Sherece. Because sometimes, growing up means facing the monsters under the bed.

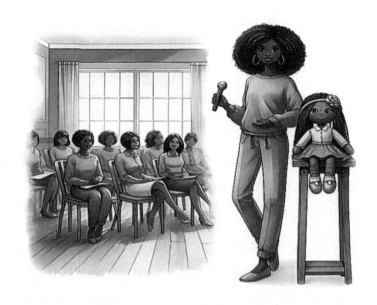

Inspired by rays of hope and the transformative power of knowledge.

Chapter Seven: From Threshold to Purpose

Tia stood poised on the threshold of her new life. The sun's golden glow embraced her as she stepped onto the stage. The graduation cap, once a mere accessory, now symbolized triumph and strength—a guide for her journey ahead. The auditorium buzzed with excitement, charged with anticipation. This graduation day held a deeper promise—a commitment etched in her heart to honor her mother's memory and carry her legacy.

As she received her certificate, Tia felt her mother's love and determination surround her. She vowed to carry this legacy with grace.

The applause echoed not only for her academic achievement but also for the silent promise she made: to be a force for change, a voice for hope. Armed with knowledge and resolve, Tia stood ready to make a difference, her journey stretching far beyond the college campus. She envisioned a world where breast cancer went beyond mere diagnosis, becoming a story of strength, empathy, recovery, and healing.

Tia's Bachelor of Science in Public Health degree became her catalyst for change. Rather than adhering to the conventional path, she veered toward hope—a winding trail through uncharted terrain. Her commitment to breast cancer awareness, education, and support propelled her mission, profoundly touching the lives of others. Her purpose extended beyond textbooks and lecture halls; it was a living force transcending boundaries.

Tia promised to be a guiding light in uncertain times. Her mother's legacy ceased to be a burden; it became a precious gift—an opportunity to ignite positive change. Even when Tia questioned her efforts, she persevered with determination. Her mother's strength resonated in her heart, and she softly replied, "Thank you, Momma. Even in suffering, there is a purpose." Tia's journey became a heartfelt tribute that combined wisdom with compassion. She knew that every step she took was a step towards honoring her mother's memory and making a difference in the world.

Tia now resided in the heart of Atlanta's historic Sweet Auburn community, where the soulful aroma of comfort food danced to jazz beats. By her side stood Tuti Tender-Heart, her cherished doll—a symbol of strength and love. Motivated by a desire to honor her mother's memory, Tia was ready and enthusiastic to raise breast cancer awareness and advocate for her community.

While Tia hadn't received a job offer directly tied to her purpose, Atlanta held compelling reasons for her choice. Sweet Auburn resonated with her vision—the rich history, soulful atmosphere, and vibrant culture provided a nurturing backdrop. Influential figures like Dr. Martin Luther King Jr. had left their mark here, inspiring Tia. She believed that by immersing herself in this vibrant city, she could amplify her efforts and create meaningful change.

Standing on the threshold of purpose, Tia sensed her mother's strength guiding her. Each step she took was a testament to the resilience she inherited. She navigated the painful twists and turns with grace, knowing they could ultimately lead to profound understanding and kindness. Her journey was not just a tribute but a living embodiment of her mother's enduring legacy.

With determination and enthusiasm, Tia began her journey in Atlanta—a place where purpose and passion met. Tuti Tender-Heart, a symbol of hope and a legacy woven from love and strength accompanied her—a torch they would pass on. As Tia and Tuti set out on their mission, her heart swelled with determination, reverence, and hope. Her mother's legacy rested gently on her shoulders, yet she remained poised and enthusiastic. Courage and love echoed within her, propelling her forward on a mission that went beyond awareness—a promise deeply rooted in her soul.

In Atlanta, Tia confronted stark truths laid bare by data. Among U.S. racial or ethnic groups, African American women faced the highest breast cancer mortality rate at 40%.[1] Shockingly, the mortality rate for Black women diagnosed with breast cancer is 42% higher than that of White women.[2] Breast cancer claims more Black lives than any other cancer.[3] Armed with this knowledge, Tia recognized the urgency to alter the narrative—a mission driven by determination and a commitment to empower women, allowing them to rewrite their stories.

With the data Tia had gathered, she hosted her first seminar on breast cancer awareness and education, naming it "Hope Blossoms: Empowering Women Against Breast Cancer." She hoped this event would motivate women to learn about prevention, early detection, and support. The seminar was held at the local community center, renowned for its commitment to breast cancer programs and events.

Tuti sat on a cushion at the front of the room, her stitched smile inviting curiosity and comfort. Tia, her wild curls bouncing and a pink ribbon gracing her blouse, greeted everyone who entered. The room buzzed with energy as women chatted, shared, and laughed. Grandmothers with colorful head wraps shared inspiring stories, while mothers cradled their little ones, eyes wide with wonder. The young women's laughter echoed as they gathered to listen— some curious, some uncertain, but all eager to discover more about breast cancer awareness and prevention.

Tia's voice trembled with emotion as she shared her mother's story of bravery, perseverance, and profound loss. She painted vivid pictures of the hardships her mother faced, yet also highlighted moments of hope that glimmered like distant stars. Her words, like seeds, took root in the receptive hearts of her audience. With compassion, she invited, "Ladies, let's engage in a conversation about our bodies—let's discuss breast health."

Tuti played a special role in the seminar, serving as a symbol of strength, love, and hope. Her presence was more than just decorative; she embodied the spirit of the event, reminding everyone of the importance of compassion and support. As Tia shared her mother's story and discussed breast cancer awareness, Tuti became a focal point for the audience, especially the younger attendees. Children were drawn to her, and she helped bridge the gap between generations, making the seminar more inclusive and engaging.

Tuti's presence also provided a gentle reminder of the personal connections and emotional bonds that drive the fight against breast cancer. Throughout the seminar, Tuti embodied the legacy Tia aimed to honor and the hope she wished to spread. Her presence inspired, comforted, and reminded everyone that love and strength could prevail despite adversity.

A touching moment during the seminar occurred when Mrs. Johnson, who had personally experienced breast cancer, stood up to share her story. With tears in her eyes, she spoke about the numerous challenges she faced and the triumphs she achieved. Despite these hardships, she found strength in her support network and community, which played a crucial role in her journey. Growing up in a small town where community and family were central to her life, Mrs. Johnson's voice wavered as she expressed gratitude for events like Tia's seminar, which provided hope and education. The room fell silent, and many attendees wiped away tears, moved by Mrs. Johnson's courage and strength. This moment underscored the importance of community and the power of shared experiences.

Tuti's petite hand directed attention to a chart on the wall, illustrating the stages of breast cancer—the silent battles waged within. Tia emphasized the significance of self-exams, early detection, and regular check-ups. As curiosity grew, the women posed a myriad of questions: "What should I do if I discover a lump?" "When is the right time for a mammogram?" "How can we safeguard our daughters?" Tia's words resonated deeply with everyone in the room. With meticulous care, she guided each woman through the essential steps of a proper self-breast check, ensuring they left with an informative illustrated pamphlet in hand.

Music played a significant role in enhancing the atmosphere of the event. Soft, uplifting melodies filled the room, creating a warm and welcoming environment. The music helped set a positive tone, making attendees feel comfortable and at ease. During breaks, lively jazz tunes brought a sense of joy and energy, encouraging conversations and connections among participants. The harmonious blend of music and heartfelt stories created an unforgettable experience, leaving everyone inspired and united in their mission to raise breast cancer awareness.

As the weeks slipped by, October—the dedicated Breast Cancer Awareness month—arrived. Tia and

Tuti took to the streets, adorning lapels, scarves, and baby strollers with pink ribbons. Their mission extended beyond symbolism; they collected donations to support women in need of mammograms. Within the heart of the African American community, they amplified their message. And there, amidst the rhythm of street drummers, Tia's melodic voice soared as she sang her song:

Know your body, sister, dear. Get the mammogram and calm your fears. Early detection is our might. Together, we will win the fight!

This powerful refrain reverberated throughout their community, kindling a flame of awareness that would shine brightly, dispelling shadows and empowering lives. As news of their mission spread, doors swung open for Tia and Tuti. Beyond the confines of Atlanta, they embarked on a journey to Birmingham and Harlem, ending at the steps of the Lincoln Memorial.

In the heart of Birmingham, local artist Beverly Denise poured her passion into a captivating mural titled "Women of Resilience." This work of art was unveiled during the special event dedicated to raising awareness about breast cancer. As Tia stood before it, she found herself drawn to the women depicted— their eyes reflecting defiance, their stories etched in scars. These were not mere brushstrokes; they were the embodiment of strength and survival.

Among the painted figures, Tia recognized faces that mirrored her journey. A woman with a headscarf, her gaze steady, symbolized the courage to face adversity head-on. Another, with hands clasped, embodied the quiet determination of caregivers who held trembling hands through the storm. And there, a silhouette dancing in the rain—a survivor who defied the odds.

Tia's fingers traced the mural's edge, sensing the pulse of countless hearts—the rhythm of determination that linked these women across time and space. Their gaze conveyed an unspoken vow: "We persist, we fight, and we rise."

Mayor Byron C. Ward extended a warm welcome to Tia, embracing her presence in their city and at the special gathering. Both personal experience and a commitment to public health inspired his deep dedication to breast cancer awareness. Witnessing his sister-in-law's battle with breast cancer profoundly influenced him, motivating his advocacy. Through community support and empowerment, Mayor Ward strove to make a difference in the fight against this disease.

Applause erupted as Tia ascended the podium. Her heart swelled with gratitude as she met his gaze, clasping his hand. "Thank you," she said, "for supporting this cause. Together, we'll create impact." Standing before the crowd, her heart raced with anticipation. She was eager to share the profound impact the foundation's work was making on countless lives throughout the Sweet Auburn community.

Tia's words resonated through the gathering, capturing everyone's attention. She spoke of determination and a shared purpose, recounting her journey—the moments of fear, the continuous support, and the victories against breast cancer. Tia leaned in, her voice earnest. "It's not just about awareness. We need to create tangible change." Faces in the crowd drew closer, their eyes reflecting understanding and empathy. Her voice carried across the square, reaching those who had faced the same battle. Tia's gratitude spilled forth—a river of appreciation for everyone who stood with them. And her closing words echoed like a powerful refrain: "Remember, we're not alone—we're united by hope."

In that moment, Birmingham became more than a city—it became a sanctuary of shared stories and the promise of brighter tomorrows. And as the gathering concluded, they lit candles—one for every survivor, every fighter, every cherished memory. The soft glow of the candles illuminated the night, symbolizing the light of hope that each person carried within them. Birmingham birthed a new anthem—a chorus of hope sung by warriors adorned in paint. The community stood together, hand in hand, their hearts beating as one, ready to face the future with renewed strength and determination.

In the vibrant heart of Harlem, Tia and Tuti actively engaged with local communities to promote breast cancer awareness. They organized and participated in workshops, heartfelt talks, and lively community events, all aimed at highlighting the importance of early detection and regular testing. Their efforts resonated deeply, inspiring hope and celebration among the brave individuals on their journey. Tuti, with her tender heart, became a symbol of support and courage, reminding everyone that they were not alone in their fight. The community came together, united by compassion and the shared goal of overcoming breast cancer, creating a network of strength and mutual support.

At the Lincoln Memorial in Washington, D.C., Tia and Tuti stood on hallowed steps. Surrounded by history, they amplified their message—breast cancer awareness, unity, and hope. Passersby listened, joining their cause. Awareness and support became shields against this relentless adversary. Their commitment went beyond mere words. Tia's melodic voice carried the refrain of her theme song:

Know your body, sister, dear. Get the mammogram and calm your fears. Early detection is our might. Together, we will win the fight!

Tia's voice united hearts in a shared purpose. Tuti, with her stitched heart, silently conveyed hope to those facing uncertainty. Together, they raised awareness, guiding others toward healing and empowerment. Their pink ribbons symbolized hope, sparking conversations everywhere. Tia encouraged women to understand their bodies, seek early detection, and support one another. In their duet of courage and compassion, Tia and Tuti created a legacy of hope, touching countless lives. They illuminated a path for their African American community and beyond.

Their travel to Birmingham, Harlem, and the Lincoln Memorial turned into a moving journey defined by understanding and a strong sense of direction. Throughout the journey, their pink ribbons, which were once purely ornamental, transformed into powerful symbols of hope, stimulating important conversations and kindling a sense of optimism. However, this was just the start—an introduction to an optimistic adventure that would lead them to destinations they had never imagined.

Tia looked back on their incredible journey as the sun went down over Sweet Auburn. "Tuti," she said, "We're not just raising awareness, we're raising hope." In that quiet moment, Tia and Tuti understood that they had become more than advocates; they were torchbearers of possibility, lighting the path for others. Like the setting sun, over their peaceful community, their legacy would linger—a reminder that hope, once kindled, could change the world.

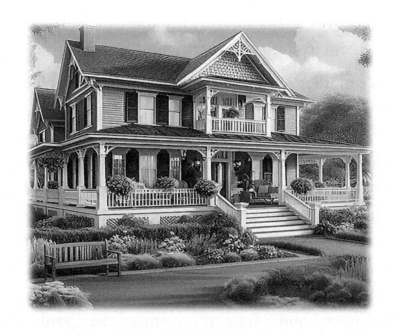

Tuti Tender-Heart Foundation
A Sanctuary of Healing, Resilience and Hope

Chapter Eight: An Unfolding Legacy

Amid the bustling city, where vibrant streets hummed with life, Tia discovered fertile soil for her vision. Pink Ribbon Unity, adorned with pink ribbons and resonating messages of hope, surpassed mere advocacy. It became a lifeline for survivors—a testament to compassion, strength, and determination.

Tia's mother's battle with breast cancer, coupled with the heartache of losing her, ignited a profound sense of empathy for Tia. She recognized that the fight against breast cancer was an immense struggle—one that no one should endure alone. With love and compassion at its core, Tia founded the Tuti Tender-Heart Foundation. The name carried a profound meaning: "Tuti" embodied resilience—the essence of hope. The foundation's mission stood firm: to empower and support women navigating the complexities of breast cancer, infusing their journey with compassion and hope. Tia's vision echoed within the hearts of those she touched, creating a legacy that would uplift and inspire generations to come.

Tia's dedication drove her tireless efforts. However, an unexpected letter changed everything. An anonymous benefactor gifted her a building—a haven nestled in a serene neighborhood. It wasn't merely property; it transformed into a canvas for healing, a sanctuary where hope could bloom.

The building stood nestled amidst whispering trees, their leaves rustling like a gentle lullaby. The scent of blooming jasmine filled the air, mingling with the earthy aroma of freshly turned soil. Sunlight streamed across the wooden floors. Inside, the walls were painted in soft, calming colors, and a nearby brook added a soothing melody to the atmosphere. This place wasn't just a building; it was a sanctuary where every corner invited peace, and every room promised comfort. Here, hope blossomed like the flowers in the garden, nurtured by the love and care of those who entered.

This place wasn't just a building; it was a sanctuary where every corner invited peace, and every room promised comfort. Here, hope blossomed like the flowers in the garden, nurtured by the love and care of those who entered.

Tia breathed life into the space where expert professionals meticulously crafted warm, inviting interiors. Counseling sessions became safe havens for sharing fears and hopes, while nutrition guidance workshops nourished both body and spirit. Expressive art therapy workshops provided survivors with a means to express their inner worlds. For those experiencing hair loss, stylish wigs and scarves adorned with heart motifs emerged as powerful reminders. These seemingly ordinary accessories transformed into symbols of renewed self-assurance. Each meticulously crafted piece reflected empathy, hope, and intention, reminding survivors that beauty lies not in hair but in the strength to face each new day.

Millie's Retreat, nestled within the grounds, flourished as a loving tribute to Tia's mother. Its winding pathway led through vibrant flowerbeds, where delicate blossoms swayed in the breeze. Sunlight filtered through leaves, dappling the ground with warmth. Amidst this natural canvas, stone benches stood, inviting quiet reflection. And there, by the small pond, the sky mirrored itself, its surface rippling gently. But it was the flowers that told stories: peonies unfurling like secrets, lavender releasing its soothing fragrance, and daffodils nodding—a reminder of strength and hope.

Each spring, survivors and supporters gathered in the serene garden, releasing delicate butterflies—a celebration of life and transformation. These winged creatures carried hope, their patterns catching sunlight and creating fleeting rainbows of color as they danced among the vibrant flowerbeds. Their flight carried the promise of change, symbolizing strength and determination.

The Tuti Tender-Heart Foundation's doors swung open on a crisp October morning, welcoming a steady stream of visitors and devoted supporters. The air buzzed with anticipation—a symphony of footsteps, hushed conversations, and eager hearts. Tia stood at the entrance, her heart brimming with gratitude. Inside this peaceful haven, visitors encountered a poignant tribute to Tia's beloved mother. The entrance featured a beautiful portrait—a heartfelt homage to the woman who had left an indelible mark on Tia's life. Beneath the portrait, a plaque overflowed with thankfulness, serving as a perpetual reminder of her mother's lasting influence. Nearby, behind glass, rested a beautifully crafted replica of the Tuti Tender-Heart doll. Its delicate features radiated compassion and love—a mirror of Tia's mother. As a living emblem of their shared legacy, it inspired all who beheld it to carry forth the spirit of kindness.

Tia's warm embrace enveloped women who had recently received a breast cancer diagnosis, cradling them in compassion. She intimately understood the gravity of their struggle—the fear, uncertainty, and fleeting moments of doubt. Her gentle words carried warmth, acknowledging the emotional rollercoaster that accompanies the battle against breast cancer. "Please know," she said softly, "that you're not alone. Within these walls lies a haven of warmth and compassion, where women like you can find solace and support." Tia's own experiences, etched with the raw emotions of her mother's battle against breast cancer, allowed her to empathize deeply with those facing similar diagnoses. Within the sanctuary's walls, her compassion became a lifeline—a powerful reminder that they were not alone in their fight.

Indeed, Tia's dream had come true. She created a sanctuary where healing and hope touched many lives. Inside, kindness thrived. Tia's smile brought comfort, encouraging people to support one another. The foundation became a special place where tears were met with compassion and laughter brought understanding. Quiet conversations shared deep experiences, and the gentle rustling of leaves echoed the strength of those seeking solace. Tia's vision turned into a living work of art, each visitor adding to a shared story of strength and connection.

"You're not alone," Tia reassured them, her voice echoing the sentiment of survivors, caregivers, and fighters. Pointing to the quilts wrapped around their shoulders, she said softly, "You are a part of this compassionate community." Her eyes reflected empathy and shared determination. Amidst the scent of herbal tea and quiet conversations, Tia saw that healing blossomed here, nurtured by vulnerability. She gently encouraged newcomers to sip chamomile tea and hold hands during chemotherapy, finding comfort in these shared moments. Beyond those walls, the world moved quickly, yet inside, time slowed. Tia's presence was a calming balm, a reminder that compassion extended beyond the confines of illness, touching hearts and inspiring hope.

Standing at the entrance, her eyes radiated gratitude and determination. The battle continued, as did hope. In Tia's serene haven, anyone seeking solace found refuge. Hope and courage were present within those walls, their rhythm echoing the promise of renewal. Each interaction—whether through shared stories, comforting touches, or quiet reassurances—unfolded strength and connection, binding hearts together. The Tuti Tender-Heart Foundation exemplified love and dedication in the fight against breast cancer. Whether newly diagnosed or long-standing warriors, visitors found reassurance within the supportive community. Tia's legacy, closely connected with her mother's, inspired perseverance and determination, guiding those navigating the turbulent waters of uncertainty.

Tia wandered through the garden, feeling the warmth of the sun on her skin and admiring the golden glow it cast on the landscape. A weathered bench, nestled beneath the ancient oak tree, held the echoes of untold stories waiting to be discovered. She settled onto it, surrounded by spring flowers whose delicate essence carried memories of Millie's love—bedtime stories, tender kisses, and the warmth of her embrace—all woven into each rose petal.

Tia let the fragrant petals transport her back in time. Millie's laughter echoed through the garden—a melody that had once filled their home. "Life," Millie would have said, "is a tapestry woven with threads of courage. Sometimes they fray, but we mend them, stitch by stitch." Tia's heart filled with both longing and determination. She remembered the nights when Millie sat on the edge of her bed, sharing tales of distant lands. The moonlight painted silver streaks across the room, and Tia's heart danced to the rhythm of her mother's words.

"You have the heart of a warrior," Millie said, brushing a kiss against Tia's forehead. "Remember that, my love." And Tia did.

When storm clouds gathered—whether as illness or adversity—she fought with the same tenacity that Millie had shown during her battle with cancer.

These memories etched themselves in Tia's mind like the veins of a leaf. Millie's wisdom echoed: courage doesn't mean you're never afraid; it means standing tall when your knees shake and finding strength in honesty.

Tia's fingers traced the rough texture of the bench. She imagined Millie sitting beside her, their hands gently touching. The ancient oak tree, wise and steadfast, seemed to nod in silent approval. "Fight, my darling," Millie's voice carried on the breeze, a gentle echo from beyond. "Fight for love, for hope, for the legacy we share." And fight she did.

Tia's memories of Millie's courage strengthened her resolve. She would lead the way for others. The Tuti Tender-Heart Foundation would flourish, its growth a promise kept. Love, like the scent of roses, lingered— a testament to a mother's enduring spirit. With every step forward, Tia felt Millie's presence guiding her, reminding her that their shared journey was far from over. The foundation would be a place where stories of triumph and perseverance would be written anew every day, offering support and inspiration to all who entered.

As the sun set, casting a warm glow over the garden, Tia made a solemn promise. She would become the dream weaver, sowing seeds of courage. The rustling leaves carried Millie's legacy—a whisper of love destined to echo through generations. Tia envisioned a future where the foundation's impact would ripple outward, touching countless lives and inspiring others to join the fight against breast cancer. In that moment, she knew that Millie's spirit would forever be a guiding light, illuminating the path toward a brighter, more hopeful tomorrow.

Beneath the ancient oak, Tia sat—a garden of memories blooming in her heart, her spirit intricately woven with threads of bravery. The whispers of the past danced around her, each one a testament to her journey. May Tia's determination and Millie's love continue to inspire, like petals carried by the wind, spreading hope and courage far and wide.

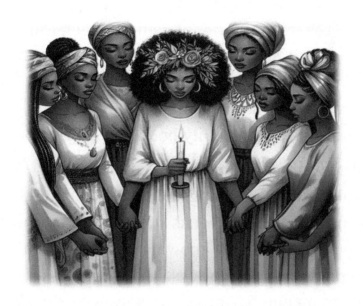

We remember. We honor. We celebrate.

Chapter Nine: Hope's Waltz

In the quiet hallways of the Tuti Tender-Heart Foundation, sunlight filtered through stained glass, casting a gentle glow upon the walls. Framed photographs and handwritten notes adorned those walls, each telling stories of battles fought, tears shed, and laughter shared. This place was more than a building; it was a refuge where survivors found solace, and warriors discovered their tribe—a compassionate community bound by empathy.

In the waiting room, where time swung like a pendulum, hope sat alongside each trembling soul. It wore no grand armor, yet its strength was unmatched. Survivors exchanged knowing glances, their eyes reflecting shared journeys. A woman, her scarf wrapped around her head like a crown, leaned in to offer hope to the newly diagnosed.

"Once, I sat where you do," she said softly. "And now look at me—a testament to hope's steadfast grace."

Her name was Lillian Harris, a retired schoolteacher. She had spent over three decades nurturing young minds and inspiring countless students with her gentle wisdom and patience. When she was diagnosed with breast cancer, Lillian faced her journey with the same grace and determination she had always shown.

Throughout her battle, she never lost her positive outlook, often sharing words of hope and encouragement with fellow patients.

After her recovery, Lillian felt a deep calling to give back to the community that had supported her. She began volunteering at the Tuti Tender-Heart Foundation, where she quickly became a cherished presence. Her experience gave her a unique ability to connect with those newly diagnosed, offering them not just advice, but genuine empathy and understanding.

Lillian connected deeply with patients, sharing her own stories of survival. She organized small gatherings for survivors to share their journeys, fostering a sense of community. In her free time, she tended to her flower garden. She enjoyed reading and writing poetry to uplift others. Her life was one of love and support, touching countless lives and leaving a lasting impact at the foundation.

Beyond the walls, the healing garden flourished. Petals unfurled, reaching eagerly for the sun. Survivors worked the soil, their hands a blend of calloused strength and gentle care. They planted seeds of hope, confident that even in winter, roots held the promise of spring. Inez, her eyes shining despite her fatigue, kneeled beside a rosebush. Her fingers gently traced the delicate petals of a rose. With a poignant look, she said, "This rose was just a bud when my treatment began. Now it blooms, and so do I."

Inez was a passionate gardener and a breast cancer survivor. Her journey through the treatment was marked by her spirit and determination. Despite the physical and emotional challenges, she found solace in the garden, where she could nurture life and witness the beauty of growth and renewal. The garden became her sanctuary, a place where she could reflect, heal, and draw strength.

Inez often shared her love for gardening with other survivors, teaching them how to care for the plants and find peace in the process. Her gentle guidance and warm presence made her a beloved figure in the community. She believed that just as the garden thrived with care and attention, so too could the human spirit flourish with hope and support.

In the chemo room, where IV lines crisscrossed, hope embraced everyone. Volunteers crocheted blankets, each stitch a prayer. "For warmth and hope," they said. Tia, despite her exhaustion, handed a blanket to a fellow warrior. "Wrap yourself in courage," she said. "You're not alone."

The chemo room was a place of quiet strength and resolve. Patients sat in comfortable chairs, their faces a mix of determination and fatigue. The soft hum of medical equipment was a constant backdrop, but it was the presence of the volunteers that brought warmth to the room. These volunteers, many of who were survivors themselves, dedicated their time to making the experience as comforting as possible.

They brought with them not just blankets, but also books, magazines, and sometimes even homemade treats. Their smiles and kind words were a balm to the weary souls undergoing treatment. Each blanket they crocheted was a symbol of solidarity and care. The volunteers often shared stories of their journeys, offering comfort and inspiration to those during their battles.

Tia, with her gentle demeanor, was a source of inspiration. Despite her exhaustion, she always found the strength to support others. Her words, "Wrap yourself in courage," were a reminder that no one had to face their journey alone. The chemo room, with its blend of medical care and heartfelt support, became a sanctuary where hope and compassion thrived.

In the foundation's hallway, a mural graced the walls—a canvas woven from survivor stories. Faces, scars, and smiles converged like threads of a vibrant quilt. Above them, the word "HOPE" stretched wide, a bridge connecting past and future. The mural, intricate and profound, etched indelible marks on visitors' hearts. As they paused, tracing the lines of courage, they heard whispers of resilience—a reminder that even amidst adversity, hope endures.

The hallway itself was a place of reflection and inspiration. Soft lighting illuminated the mural, casting gentle shadows that seemed to dance with the stories depicted. Benches lined the walls, inviting visitors to sit and absorb the powerful messages. Plaques beneath the mural shared brief narratives of individuals portrayed, adding depth to their visual stories. The air was filled with a quiet reverence as if the very walls held the collective strength of those who had walked this path.

Beneath the mural, a framed handwritten letter spoke with sincerity:

To those who held my hand during the storm, you were my lighthouse in the tempest. Your smiles, like bright lights, guided me through the darkest nights. Thank you for stitching hope into my veins, for whispering courage when my heart faltered. Your constant support and kindness were the anchors that kept me grounded. Each day, I carry your love with me, a beacon that lights my path forward. With love and eternal gratitude. ~ Jasmine

On the anniversary of Millie's passing, the foundation gathered. Candles flickered, casting shadows on tear-streaked faces. Tia stepped forward, her voice steady. "We remember and we honor. But let us also celebrate. Hope persists—it's part of our legacy. Each survivor, each story, each act of kindness—these create a legacy of compassion. Today, let our tears meet with gratitude, and our grief finds solace in the promise of brighter days."

This gathering was important for various reasons. It was an opportunity to commemorate and honor Millie, whose life and battle with breast cancer led to the establishment of the foundation. Her memory served as an inspiration, reminding everyone of the importance of early detection and the strength of community support in the fight against breast cancer.

Tia's words emphasized the importance of celebrating hope and determination. Despite the grief and loss, the gathering highlighted the enduring spirit of those who continued to fight and support each other. This gathering was not just a memorial but a celebration of life, hope, and the enduring power of community. It was a poignant reminder that even in the face of loss, there is always room for gratitude and the promise of a better future.

As the sun set, survivors joined hands in the garden, forming a circle. Their voices blended—a chorus of gratitude, grief, and hope. Tomorrow wasn't just another day; it was a garden waiting for blossoms, nurtured by hearts fluent in the language of possibility.

In this sacred space, hope blossomed, transcending grief. Their unified strength declared, "We remember, we honor, and we celebrate—for hope blooms eternal."

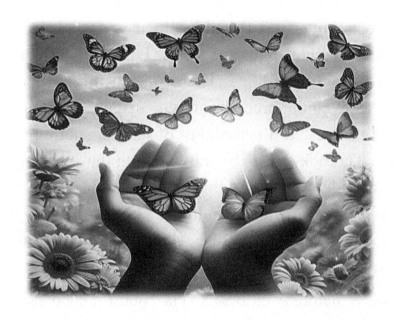

Hope, akin to butterflies, knows no limits.

Chapter Ten: Whispers of Hope

Tia settled into a cozy chair on the front porch, her gaze tracing the tranquil expanse of the Tuti Tender-Heart Foundation's grounds. As the sun dipped below the horizon, it cast a warm glow on the flower beds. Delicate butterflies flitted by, their wings adorned in iridescent blues and soft pinks. Each flutter seemed like a promise of hope. The gentle rustling of leaves in the evening breeze and the distant chirping of crickets created a symphony of nature, soothing her soul. Tia took a deep breath, inhaling the sweet scent of lavender and roses that filled the air. She felt a sense of peace and gratitude, knowing that this sanctuary was a place of healing and renewal for so many.

Amidst nature's embrace, Tia found solace as she cradled Tuti close to her heart. The doll's stitches held stories of resilience, much like the women who sought refuge at the foundation. Tuti, this cherished gift, had been a source of comfort during Tia's darkest days. As she gently held the doll, memories of her mother's love and courage flooded her mind, bringing a bittersweet smile to her lips. The soft fabric of Tuti seemed to absorb her worries, leaving behind a sense of calm and hope. Tia knew that, just like the flowers in the garden, she too would continue to grow and bloom, nurtured by the love and support of those around her.

Tia closed her eyes, recalling the moment when Millie placed Tuti in her hands. She remembered the delicate details on Tuti's fabric features: the bright eyes, the stitched smile, and the delicate pink heart on her chest. Millie's voice echoed in Tia's mind: "This is Tuti Tender-Heart, your special doll. Tuti carries hope and comfort. Even in the toughest moments, there's always hope. Hold her close when I'm gone; she'll remind you of my love." At that moment, Tia had wondered, "How can a doll be so special?" But as time went by, she understood just how true her mother's words were. Indeed, Tuti had been that to her and so much more.

A tender-hearted gift from her mother, Tuti stood faithfully by Tia's side throughout her journey. Her hand-drawn eyes held secrets—the shared laughter during chemotherapy sessions, promises exchanged in hospital rooms, and tears shed when hope seemed elusive. With a stitched mouth that curved into both a smile and poignant sadness, Tuti, the cloth doll, had become an integral part of their mission: a sanctuary for women facing breast cancer. In her silent presence, Tuti carried hope like a fragile butterfly, fluttering alongside the survivors.

Tuti was more than just a doll; she was a symbol of enduring love and strength. Each time Tia held her, she felt a connection to her mother, as if Millie's comforting presence was still with her. The doll's soft fabric absorbed Tia's fears and worries, bringing a sense of calm and reassurance. Tuti's presence was a reminder that even in the darkest times, there was always a glimmer of hope.

As Tia and the foundation continued their work, Tuti became a source of comfort for other women. Passed around during support group meetings, her stitched smile offered solace to those who needed it most. The women shared their stories, drawing strength from each other and Tuti's silent support. The doll's journey mirrored their own, filled with moments of joy and sorrow.

In the garden, where flowers bloomed and butterflies danced, Tuti was a constant companion. She sat on benches during quiet moments of reflection and was held close during celebrations. Tuti's presence was a testament to the power of love and the unbreakable bond between mother and daughter, symbolizing the foundation's mission to provide hope, comfort, and support to all who walked through its doors.

At Millie's Retreat, survivors found solace in a tranquil haven. Within the foundation's serene setting, they openly shared their stories, gathering in circles where their voices harmonized like sacred hymns. Each scar transformed into a badge of honor, every tear a testament to fortitude. Tia listened, her heart swelling with pride. These women, warriors in their battles, wove hope into life's fabric. Together, they carried Tia's legacy forward, their pink-embroidered hearts beating in unison.

Among the survivors, some bloomed anew after the storm. They danced like confetti in the wind, their laughter filling the hallways. Tia marveled at their strength—the way they found joy even in the darkest times. They proved that hope wasn't just a concept; it was a lifeline, shared heart-to-heart. In her mind's eye, Tia saw Millie dancing among them, her spirit entwined with those she had loved and lost.

The butterfly release ceremony symbolized transformation—a poignant reminder that hope could emerge from the darkest corners of existence. During the ceremony, participants would release butterflies into the garden. This act represented the journey from struggle to renewal, mirroring the experiences of those supported by the foundation. It was a beautiful and moving tribute to resilience and the enduring spirit of hope.

The ink dried on the parchment, and Tia stood before the foundation's mural. She traced her life's journey and the profound impact she'd made. The artwork depicted Millie and fellow warriors who had faced similar adversaries.

Tia's fingers outlined the pink heart on Tuti's chest, pausing at the stitches. "Dear Tuti," she said, "we've come a long way. Your tender heart lives on in every survivor, in every shared story. And Millie, your legacy transcends these walls—it's woven into life's very fabric."

Outside, stars blinked like distant candles in the night sky. Tia closed her eyes, feeling the weight of the journey—the losses, the victories, and the love that had sustained her. Knowing she hadn't faced the journey alone, she said, "Tuti, you're more than a doll. You're a ray of hope, intricately woven into our legacy.

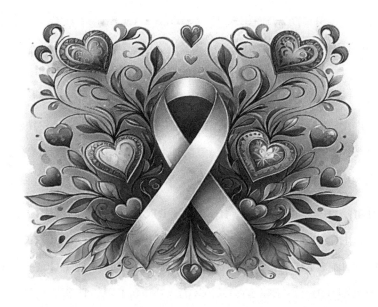

Resilience and hope — a mural of hearts,
each thread weaving stories of survival.

Chapter Eleven: Echoes of Recognition

Nestled at the crossroads of hope and healing, the Tuti Tender-Heart Foundation radiated its impact outward like gentle waves on a tranquil pond. Recognition arrived unexpectedly—first through a feature in the local newspaper where the stories of survivors and the foundation's compassionate work took center stage. The article eloquently captured the transformative effect of hope within the community, stating, "Today, we share Velma's remarkable journey—a survivor forever touched by the support of the Tuti Tender-Heart Foundation."

Velma, once vibrant, faced a breast cancer diagnosis that changed her life. With no job, home, or immediate family, she turned to the Tuti Tender-Heart Foundation. Their swift, compassionate response was profoundly impactful. Beyond emotional support, they gifted her a cloth doll—a symbol of survival. Velma shared that Tuti's heart, stitched into the fabric, held hope, reminding her she was not alone in her fight.

The foundation's counselors stayed by Velma's side, guiding her through uncertainty with practical support. They provided financial aid, arranged transportation, and ensured her focus remained on healing. In support groups, Velma found solace and a healing atmosphere—a lifeline when she needed it most.

Velma's uncertainty gave way to the foundation's compassionate care. Through chemotherapy, she gained new insights and hope. The consistent support transformed her journey, turning doubt into strength. Velma emerged not just as a survivor but as an inspiration to others facing similar challenges.

The support groups profoundly impacted Velma, offering a safe space to express her fears and hopes without judgment. Surrounded by those who understood her journey, she felt a deep sense of belonging and acceptance. The shared stories and mutual encouragement empowered her, providing the strength to face each chemotherapy session. These connections became a vital source of comfort and motivation, helping her navigate the emotional highs and lows of her treatment.

Inspired by the foundation's tender heart, Velma vowed to give back. She became an advocate, spreading hope and compassion. Today, Velma is a testament to the foundation's impact, reminding us that compassion can bloom even in dark times. The foundation's ripple effect continues, touching lives far beyond our city limits.

Reflecting on her experience, Velma shared, "The Tuti Tender-Heart Foundation gave me more than just support; they gave me a family. Their love and care turned my darkest days into a journey of hope and strength. I am forever grateful and committed to paying it forward."

Next came an interview at a prominent television station. Tia, the driving force behind the foundation, sat down to share her vision, hope, and the heartbeat of their mission. Her words transcended borders, inspiring countless viewers to join the cause and become part of the legacy of compassion.

As survivors' testimonies echoed through the foundation, its impact grew even stronger.

Amidst the serene quiet of the foundation's library, Tia sat down when a letter arrived. Its contents promised to add another poignant chapter to the story of hope and compassion she had lovingly cultivated. The letter bore the official seal of the Mayor's office, and Tia's trembling hands unfolded its message. It began with heartfelt words: "In recognition of outstanding service to our community." The Tuti Tender-Heart Foundation received the prestigious Heart of Compassion Award.

The celebratory ceremony on the foundation's grounds brought together staff members, and community supporters—a heartfelt gathering that emphasized the dedication Tia and her team had poured into their mission. Survivors expressed their gratitude through tearful smiles, heartfelt words, and clenched hands. Some shared personal stories of strength and perseverance, while others simply embraced Tia, their eyes reflecting the depth of their appreciation.

The ceremony reverberated with a shared sense of unity—an acknowledgment that they hadn't journeyed alone. Applause erupted, and tears flowed as Tuti sat proudly on the podium, watching the Mayor himself present the award and shake Tia's hand. Cameras flashed, capturing the moment—the intersection of grief and triumph stitched together like Tuti's heart.

As the applause subsided, Tia stepped forward to address the gathering. "Ladies and gentlemen, esteemed guests, thank you for being here today," she began. "When we founded the Tuti Tender-Heart Foundation, our mission was simple: to bring hope into the lives of women battling breast cancer. Little did we realize that our compassion would extend beyond walls and boundaries. Our foundation goes beyond providing medical aid; it's about transforming life's challenges—fear, pain, and uncertainty—into something beautiful. Millie's legacy thrives in every heart here, reminding us that together, we can overcome anything and blossom with renewed strength and hope."

Tia's gaze shifted to Tuti, who sat beside her, pride shining in her eyes. From childhood to the foundation's inception, Tuti had been a steadfast presence—a source of strength during tough times. Together, they navigated challenges, celebrated victories, and shared stories that painted a canvas of courage. The audience leaned in, captivated by Tia's words. She recounted stories of survivors: a girl who painted flowers and rainbows on hospital walls, a woman who danced despite chemotherapy, and a mother who sang lullabies to her child during treatment. Their resilience became the bedrock of the foundation.

"And today," Tia declared, her voice steady, "we receive recognition not for ourselves but for the countless lives touched by our work. The whispers of hope have grown into a strong chorus, reaching far and wide. Our efforts have connected communities and hearts with shared determination. I am deeply grateful for each one of you who has been part of this journey."

As Tia descended from the podium, the applause still echoing in her ears, Tuti leaned in and said, "You've done it; Millie would be so proud." Tia's eyes welled up with tears. "We're the weavers of hope," she replied. "Together, we'll keep stitching until every heart finds solace."

With the applause and flashing cameras surrounding her, Tia understood the importance of this moment. She saw the result of many hours of hard work, dedication, and shared compassion. Through this journey, Tia had grown immensely, finding her strength and purpose. The Tuti Tender-Heart Foundation was a place of hope, offering comfort to those in need. Cancer would no longer be fought alone; it would meet understanding and support. Tia looked at Tuti and said, "Our journey has been long, my friend. Millie's legacy isn't just within these walls; it's part of humanity."

As evening fell, Tia and Tuti stood before a mural of embroidered hearts, each telling a survivor's story of pain, healing, and hope. Reflecting on the day, Tia said, "This mural is more than art. It's a testament to hope, created by hands that have known both struggle and renewal." Later, in the soft glow of the mural, Tia and Tuti sat together. Tuti said, "To us, this mural is more than hearts. We're part of this story, shaped by compassion." Tia nodded, her eyes tracing the delicate stitches. "Echoes of recognition," she said proudly. "That's what we are, Tuti."

In the quiet of that moment, they realized their role: storytellers. They weren't merely observers; they were creators of a legacy—a legacy of love. They were crafting stories of love, hope, and perseverance. Each piece was a part of their shared experiences, capturing moments of joy, sorrow, and triumph. These stories were not just about the past but also about inspiring future generations to cherish and continue the legacy of compassion and connection.

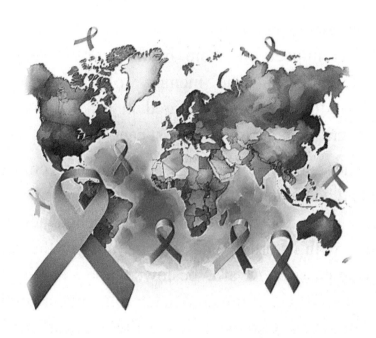

Celebrating the power of unity and interconnected hearts.

Chapter Twelve: Threads Across Continents

Tia's journey extended far beyond geographical boundaries. Her heart was a map of interconnected threads of compassion and determination. What had once begun as a small, local endeavor, the Tuti Tender-Heart Foundation now spanned continents, with its impact felt from bustling city centers to remote villages. The memory of the Heart of Compassion Award glimmered in Tia's mind as a testament to their tireless breast cancer support work.

With her compassionate heart and boundless empathy, Tia had dedicated her life to supporting those battling breast cancer, a disease that had touched her own family with its cruel hand. The memory of the Heart of Compassion Award, bestowed upon her by the Mayor's Office, glimmered in her mind like a guiding star. It was a testament to the tireless work of the foundation and its volunteers, who labored diligently to provide comfort, care, and healing to those in need.

Tia carried within her the stories of countless individuals whose lives had been touched by the foundation's work. Each face, each voice, was etched into her memory, fueling her resolve to continue fighting for those who needed support.

The Tuti Tender-Heart Foundation reached diverse communities, offering support and resources where they were needed most. From organizing health camps in rural areas to hosting awareness events in major cities, the foundation's presence grew stronger. Volunteers from different parts of the world joined hands, united by a common goal. Each project, each story shared, added to the growing network of support and empowerment.

As the invitations arrived, Tia opened each one with care. Some invited her to share her story at international conferences, while others extended collaboration invitations for global initiatives. Each envelope held the promise of bringing together a community of hope, connecting hearts across borders.

Tia marveled at the diversity of the requests—an invitation to speak at a medical symposium in Tokyo, a call to join a panel on women's health in Nairobi, and a proposal for a collaborative project with a foundation in Buenos Aires. Each letter was a testament to the growing impact of the Tuti Tender-Heart Foundation. Tia felt a profound sense of purpose as she envisioned the countless lives that could be touched through these opportunities. The world was opening up, and with it, the chance to spread their message of love and support even further.

Hope, like a universal melody, transcended cultural boundaries. Across those borders, hearts beat in unison, echoing the rhythm of survival. The Tuti Tender-Heart doll, once a humble symbol, now stood tall as an Ambassador of Hope, weaving connections between cultures, spanning oceans, and leaving its tender mark on lives across the globe.

In Mumbai, amidst fragrant air and bustling markets, Tia and Tuti Tender-Heart carried hope. They ventured into vibrant neighborhoods, where the doll embodied courage. Children clung to it, their eyes reflecting unwavering determination—the same resolve that fueled Tia's mission. Across the sun-kissed savannah of Kenya, the doll transformed into Kenya's Ambassador of Hope. It journeyed to remote villages, offering solace and strength. Survivors huddled beneath acacia trees, sharing tales of survival. The doll listened, its stitched heart absorbing their pain and echoing their triumphs.

These journeys and the stories they gathered along the way were immortalized in the mural back home at the foundation. The mural's stitches held stories of bravery, loss, and love. Tia found herself at the heart of a cultural crossroads. Symbolizing unity, her heart pulsed with the rhythm of interconnectedness. As she meticulously added stitches to the mural, Tia's words resonated with a profound truth that transcended physical boundaries. Each thread became a bridge, linking people across countries—demonstrating the resilience of the human spirit.

Immortalized in the mural, Millie's legacy reached far beyond city limits. It transcended oceans, languages, and time zones, binding people together in a shared journey of love and strength—a symphony of empathy and understanding. Tia, gazing at the intricate patterns, felt awe at the human connection. The fabric spoke of triumph over adversity, revealing unbreakable bonds between souls separated by vast distances. Each stitch seemed to breathe life into the mural, echoing whispers of encouragement, shared laughter, and tears from those who had walked similar paths. As she stood there, surrounded by the collective heartbeat of determination, Tia knew that this mural was more than art—it was a testament to the enduring spirit of humanity.

Tia's thoughts flowed through the threads of memory as she stood before the mural. Her mother, Millie, had battled breast cancer—a fierce struggle that ignited this remarkable journey. But the mural was more than a tribute; it stood as a symbol of hope, casting its colors across countless lives.

Each thread held a story—a survivor's strength, a supporter's steadfast commitment. Woven together like a global quilt, the fabric resonated with diverse experiences. Tia's finger traced the stitches, and in that touch, she felt the pulse of a vast community— the foundation's enduring legacy.

Despite oceans and borders, they were bound by purpose. The mural breathed life into their shared mission, bridging distances with love and solidarity. It whispered, "You are not alone."

Tia's purpose rekindled. The foundation's work was compassion crystallized—a promise etched in every stitch. For her mother, for all mothers, she vowed to fight on. Each thread became a lifeline, connecting hearts across continents.

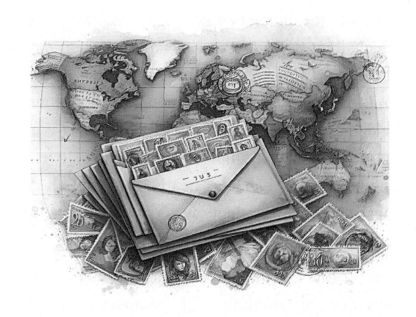

Threads of compassion connecting distant lands.

Chapter Thirteen: Threads of Compassion

In the tranquil sunroom of the foundation, Tia sat by the window, her gaze drawn to the raindrops outside. Childhood memories, delicate as threads, wove through her emotions. The lingering scent of chamomile tea enveloped her—a warm balm against life's challenges. Millie, as a steadfast anchor, played an essential role in Tia's life. Even when Tia was young, Millie's constant support and courage provided stability during difficult times. Like an anchor that holds a ship steady, Millie's love and strength anchored Tia's heart, allowing her to navigate life's turbulent waters with hope and determination.

Millie profoundly influenced Tia. She taught her the importance of strength and compassion through stories of kindness. Millie's gentle guidance and belief in Tia instilled confidence and purpose. During her battle with breast cancer, Millie's bravery and positive spirit inspired Tia. Her constant smile and encouraging words became Tia's source of strength.

Millie's influence went beyond emotional support. She nurtured Tia's curiosity and creativity, encouraging her to explore the world with an open heart and mind. They spent hours crafting, reading, and dreaming about the future. These moments built the foundation of Tia's compassionate nature and her drive to make a difference.

As Tia grew older, Millie's legacy continued to shape her path. The lessons of love, courage, and empathy that Millie taught became the guiding principle of the Tuti Tender-Heart Foundation. Tia's work was a tribute to her mother's enduring spirit and their unbreakable bond.

Millie's beloved song played in Tia's mind, reminding her of love and endurance. The melody mixed with the rain tapping on the glass, creating a symphony of memories. Tia felt her mother's legacy—the battles fought, woven into her being. In that moment, her heart held both ache and gratitude, connecting past and present.

Tia's mind rewound to their quiet promises—the late-night conversations, the shared laughter, and the Tuti Tender-Heart doll cradled in her arms. She could almost feel the warmth of Millie's hands as she placed the doll in Tia's grasp, whispering, "For hope—to remind you forever of my love." Even in the darkest hours, a delicate thread of light persisted, weaving its way through their hearts.

The journey began in the sterile doctor's office, where the truth about breast cancer hung heavy in the air, mixed with the antiseptic scent. Tia stood there, determined, making a promise to her mother. She pledged to bring hope to every heart, just as Millie had filled their lives with love. The memory of that promise, made in Dr. Sherece's office, was etched in Tia's mind. Each stitch she sewed and every word she spoke carried their legacy forward—a testament to compassion, hope, and their unbreakable bond.

Tia and Tuti embarked on their journey together. The Tuti Tender-Heart doll, with its stitched heart, became her silent friend, witnessing chemotherapy sessions, prayers, and tearful nights. Tuti's cloth arms held pain, fear, and strength that grew in adversity. The smell of hospital disinfectant, the hum of machines, and the soft rustle of Tuti's fabric against Tia's cheek were the backdrop of their story.

As the seasons passed, the Tuti Tender-Heart Foundation became a sanctuary for survivors—a place where they found comfort and shared their stories. Tia's vision reached beyond local boundaries, gaining nationwide recognition. The Heart of Compassion Award on the office wall reflected their achievements and commitment to strength and empathy. Within those walls, survivors found solace and a sisterhood—an interconnected network built on shared experiences and the belief that compassion could heal deep wounds.

The sisterhood thrived—a resilient tapestry of shared experiences. These women, united by their battles with breast cancer, leaned on one another. They shared stories of courage, vulnerability, and survival. In whispered conversations, they found comfort, understanding, and the strength to face each day. Together, they turned adversity into a shared journey—a testament to the bond that transcended illness.

Invitations arrived now from around the world—letters from distant lands. Some asked about the foundation's work, while others urgently sought support. Japan, India, and Kenya invited the Tuti Tender-Heart Foundation to establish programs in their countries. Tia felt the weight of spreading hope across borders and fostering compassion in new communities. These global connections reminded her that compassion transcended boundaries, and Millie's love reached far beyond their local haven.

Tia stood at a crossroads, carefully opening letters from three nations. Each invitation was an opportunity to expand the foundation's mission internationally. She imagined the survivors in those far-off places: their quiet prayers, bravery, and longing for comfort. These letters carried the hopes and dreams of communities across borders, uniting hearts in a shared purpose and determination.

Tia embraced her mission, rallying her team of tireless volunteers, survivors who felt like family, and Dr. Delreeco, their steadfast supporter. His concern for people affected by breast cancer brought him to the foundation, where he combined medical expertise with compassion. Together, they wove a fabric of hope, determination, and commitment, touching lives across borders. Tia admired how Dr. Delreeco listened to both symptoms and the stories in each survivor's eyes. For him, medicine was a link between science and the human spirit, echoing hope throughout the foundation's corridors.

Together the team charted a global vision for the foundation. Their plan included hosting tea ceremonies in Japan, blending tradition with healing conversations. The fragrant steam rising from porcelain cups would carry whispers of solace, bridging hearts across generations. In India, colorful threads would weave through support circles, connecting people across languages and cultures. These threads, like the intricate patterns of a sari, would bind souls together, creating a fabric of understanding and empathy. In Kenya, under the vast African sky, they would plant seeds—nurturing them with both the strength of the earth and the unity of the community. Each seedling would stretch its roots toward the sun, mirroring the determination of those who tended to it. As Tuti rested on the windowsill, her heart, stitched in pink, seemed to affirm their shared purpose, echoing the spirit of those they served.

Tia's mother's voice echoed: "Love knows no boundaries, my dear." With renewed determination, Tia penned her responses to the invitations. The Tuti Tender-Heart Foundation would stretch its arms wide, embracing survivors across oceans. Once stitched by Millie's hands, the quilt of hope would now span continents.

As the rain gently tapped on the window, Tia reflected, "Mom, we're weaving a blanket of courage—one that spans distance and disease. Our strands of love will wrap around hearts in Tokyo, Mumbai, and Nairobi. She envisioned Millie present, saying, "Carry it forward."

Millie's spirit lingered in Tia's memory like a precious thread sewn into the fabric of her existence. With pride, Millie would have followed the threads of compassion, seeing the legacy left by Tia—a story of hope that crosses national boundaries.

In the quiet corridors, Tia listened. She heard the strength in those whispers, the echoes of survival. Each branch of the Tuti Tender-Heart Foundation became a symphony—a melody of compassion that transcended borders. Tia's steady heartbeat conducted this global mission. She understood that hope was the universal language, and courage its sweet refrain.

As Tia leaves the foundation, her heart swells with a mix of emotions. She knows this journey is vital for the global vision her team created. Thinking about the lives touched by the Tuti Tender-Heart Foundation, Tia feels connected to the survivors and families. With Tuti nestled in her bag, she is reminded of her mission and the love that drives her. Tia is optimistic, believing her journey will create new connections and spread compassion worldwide.

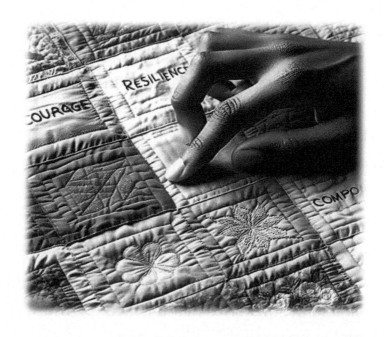

Healing Stitches, Timeless Love

Chapter Fourteen: Threads of Eternity

Tia's return flight was comfortable, though she was tired from her journey. At the terminal, her nephew Chase awaited her with a big smile and a warm hug. After graduating, Chase moved to Atlanta, touched by Tia's invitation. He felt honored and excited to join the Tuti Tender-Heart Foundation. Inspired by Millie's memory and the foundation's mission, he was determined to make a meaningful impact. Working closely with Aunt Tia and the women they supported, he found the perfect opportunity to contribute significantly.

"Welcome back, Aunt Tia! How was the trip?" Chase asked, his eyes sparkling with curiosity.

"It was enlightening, Chase. I met so many incredible women and heard stories that touched my heart," Tia replied, her voice filled with warmth.

As they walked to the car, Chase continued, "I can't wait to hear all about it. Did you get a chance to visit any of the new breast cancer support centers?"

"Yes, and they were even more amazing than I imagined. The women there are so resilient and inspiring. It reminded me why we started this journey in the first place," Tia said, her eyes misting with emotions.

Chase nodded, understanding the depth of her feelings. "You've done something truly remarkable, Aunt Tia. The foundation is changing lives every day."

Tia smiled, "And you're a big part of that, Chase. Your dedication means the world to me and to everyone we help."

Chase blushed slightly, "I'm just following your lead. You've always been my inspiration."

They reached the car, and as Chase loaded Tia's luggage into the trunk, he asked, "So what's next on the agenda for the foundation?"

Tia thought for a moment, "We're planning a new outreach program to connect with younger women. Early detection and support are crucial, and we want to make sure they have all the resources they need."

"That sounds fantastic. How can I help?" Chase asked eagerly.

"There's plenty to do. We'll need to organize events, create educational materials, and reach out to communities. Your tech skills will be invaluable for our online campaigns," Tia said.

Chase grinned, "I'm on it. Let's make this the best program yet."

As they drove home, Tia's mind wandered between gratitude and reflection. She thought about the countless lives touched by the Tuti Tender-Heart Foundation. Sitting comfortably in the cozy corner of the foundation's library later that evening, she let the memories wash over her. The foundation has made a significant difference, both in the community and worldwide.

The warm greeting from Dr. Delreeco earlier that day served as a poignant reminder of the far-reaching influence her journey had, and the ever-growing legacy of hope she had established. The oncologist's eyes, filled with compassion, revealed their profound understanding. "Tia," he said, "the impact of your work is deep and far-reaching."

Tia smiled, feeling a renewed sense of purpose. She knew that the threads of eternity were woven through every act of kindness, every moment of resilience, and every story of hope that the foundation has inspired. "Dr. Delreeco," she replied, "we're creating a tapestry of hope, just like this quilt here in our library. Each stitch represents courage, compassion, and hope."

Her fingers moved along the embroidered quilt, a collection of memories stitched together. Each square held meaning: vibrant pink for courage, soft blue for strength, and delicate lace for compassion. Millie's stitches, woven during her breast cancer battle, carried love and strength.

Dr. Delreeco leaned against the doorframe, his voice filled with excitement as he addressed Tia. "Tia," he said, "I'm thrilled about the developments here. But let's give you some rest before I share our latest report."

Tia's gentle smile conveyed more than words ever could. As she gazed out the window, the distant birds' songs and the soft rustling of leaves filled the air, drawing her mother closer to her heart. She imagined the comforting hand on her shoulder and the silent encouragement to persevere. Tia remembered the letter that her mother had written her before she passed away. These words resonated: *"Tia, your dreams are like stars in the night sky. Reach for them. Imagine far-off lands and adventures carried by the wind. Dream until your heart overflows with possibility. Your heart, a treasure chest of courage and wonder, holds the keys to countless doors. Open them fearlessly."*

Reflecting on her mother's words, Tia felt pride and determination. She had visited far-off lands, just as her mother had envisioned. The vibrant culture of Japan, the rich traditions of India, and the breathtaking landscapes of Kenya had all left an indelible mark on her heart.

During her journey in Kenya, Tia experienced a memorable encounter that would stay with her forever. She was visiting a small village where the Tuti Tender-Heart Foundation had recently established a community center. The center provided support and resources for women battling breast cancer, offering a safe space for them to share their stories and find strength in each other.

One afternoon, Tia was invited to join a gathering of women at the center. As she entered the room, she was greeted with warm smiles and the sound of laughter. The women, dressed in vibrant, colorful fabrics, were seated in a circle, sharing their experiences and offering words of encouragement. Tia took a seat among them, feeling a deep sense of connection.

One woman, named Elinah, stood up to speak. She was a breast cancer survivor and an inspiration to the community. Elinah's eyes lit up as she talked about her journey, from being diagnosed to finishing her treatment. As Elinah spoke, Tia was drawn to a small girl sitting beside her, clutching a handmade doll. The doll had a kind face and a heart stitched on its chest, reminiscent of Tuti Tender-Heart. Tia's heart warmed as she remembered how Tuti had comforted her during Millie's treatments, providing solace during the most challenging times.

Elinah introduced the girl as her daughter, Zawadi, and explained how the doll had been a source of comfort for Zawadi during her mother's treatments. Tia was not just moved by Elinah and Zawadi's story but by each story shared during the gathering of women at the center. Moved by their stories, Tia felt tears welling up in her eyes. She realized that the foundation's work was about providing resources and creating a sense of community and hope. Elinah's strength and Zawadi's constant support were a testament to the power of love and courage.

After the gathering, Elinah approached Tia and handed her a small, intricately woven bracelet. "This is for you," Elinah said, her voice filled with gratitude. "It's a symbol of our bond and the hope you've brought to our village."

Tia accepted the bracelet with a heartfelt smile, feeling a profound sense of fulfillment. This encounter reinforced her commitment to the foundation's mission and reminded her of the incredible impact that even the smallest acts of kindness could have. As she left the village, Tia looked back at the community center, now bustling with life and laughter. She knew that the threads of hope they had joined together would continue to strengthen and grow, connecting hearts across the world. Each place she visited had taught her something new about hope and the power of community.

The library's quiet ambiance provided the perfect backdrop for Tia's thoughts. The shelves, filled with books and artifacts from around the world, were a testament to the foundation's global reach. Tia's eyes landed on a globe in the corner, and she traced her recent travels with her finger, feeling a deep connection to each place. Her gaze then shifted to a framed photograph on the wall. It was a picture of her mother, Millie, smiling warmly with Tuti Tender-Heart in her arms. The doll, with its kind eyes and gentle smile, had truly become a symbol of the foundation's mission. Tia felt a wave of gratitude for her mother's legacy.

With a renewed sense of purpose, Tia stood up and walked over to the quilt. She gently touched the squares, feeling the textures of courage, strength, and compassion. Each stitch was a reminder of the countless lives touched by the foundation's work. She knew that her journey was far from over, and there were still many doors to open.

As the sun began to set, casting a warm glow through the library windows, Tia made a silent promise to herself. She would continue to dream, to reach for the stars, and to carry her mother's legacy forward. With every step she took, she would weave threads of hope, courage, and love into the fabric of the world.

The beautiful therapeutic artwork that covered the walls appeared to be surging with life, with each brushstroke expressing a tale of perseverance. Her heart grew proud and humbled at the same time. She could very clearly recall the first woman who had trembled through their doors, dread giving way to growing optimism. With a scarcely audible voice, Tia added, "Mom, we're making an impact. More hearts are healed by your love and stitches than we could have ever dreamed."

As the warm rays of the afternoon sun enveloped the quilt, Tia realized that these strands of love and hope would reach countless generations, uniting survivors in a comforting embrace of strength. Each stitch, carefully placed, represented the very essence of hope. This legacy transcended time, whispering encouragement to those yet to face their battles.

Much like the Tuti Tender-Heart Foundation, the quilt held stories of survival, compassion, and support. Tuti, the cloth doll, embodied hope—a guiding light for those navigating the turbulent waters of illness. And with each sincere conversation, Dr. Delreeco, the foundation's dedicated oncologist, stood alongside survivors, giving them hope. The foundation's mission spread compassion worldwide, creating a global network of courage. Tia, inspired by her mother's legacy, knew that true strength was about bringing hope into every aspect of life.

In the quiet library, Tia's gaze shifted toward Tuti, who sat by the window—a gentle reminder of her mother's love and the foundation's purpose. Love, hope, and the legacy of both Millie and Tuti Tender-Heart connected survivors in an eternal embrace.

And so, dear reader, as the final chapter draws to a close, remember that Hope has no boundaries. It dwells in survivors' hearts, and it keeps us moving forward. Hope echoes through the corridors of the foundation, binding a mother, her daughter, and a cloth doll named Tuti Tender-Heart in an unbreakable bond.

May Tuti Tender-Heart's Journey of Hope and Tia and Millie's legacy forever inspire us. Let the Tuti Tender-Heart Foundation remain a sanctuary where hope and healing abound. As you close this chapter, carry this legacy forward, nurturing it—one heartbeat at a time.

Tia's phone buzzed—an incoming message from Dr. Delreeco. The words on the screen read, "We've secured a grant for breast cancer research, and your mother's name is on it." Tears filled Tia's eyes as she typed her reply: "Thank you, Dr. Delreeco. Millie's legacy lives on."

In hearts that beat with love so true,
A mission born a dream pursued.
Through trials faced and battles won,
Hope and courage shine as one.

With Tuti's touch and Tia's grace,
Compassion spreads from place to place.
Together, hand in hand we stand,
To heal, to love, across the land.

Spreading Hope and Love
One Heart At A Time

EPILOGUE

Vigilance and Victory: Embracing the Journey Beyond Breast Cancer

Approximately one in eight women globally are impacted by breast cancer. While prevention isn't guaranteed, it is crucial to equip women with the tools to navigate these challenges. Regular screenings and check-ups empower individuals to take charge of their health, increasing the chances of early detection. Early detection is key to successful treatment and recovery.

The steady beat of the human heart symbolizes our ability to endure adversity and emerge stronger. This strength underscores the importance of maintaining breast cancer vigilance year-round, beyond October. Early detection significantly increases survival rates, but it is not just about medical screenings; emotional support and empathy are vital too. Offering comfort and understanding through kind words and gestures bolsters mental health.

Education is a powerful shield, providing essential knowledge to recognize early signs of disease. This awareness empowers swift responses and effective strategies to control illnesses, guiding us toward optimal health and a promising future.

And let us never forget the survivors, the warriors who have faced adversity and emerged victorious. Their victories inspire hope for those still fighting their battles. In life's journey, we find strength. Breast cancer may surprise us, but remember, you're not alone. You're stronger than you think–you're a fighter, full of hope. Each scar, each tear, and each moment of steadfast courage connect hearts across continents. Together, we stand—a global sisterhood bound by compassion, tenacity, and unshakable hope.

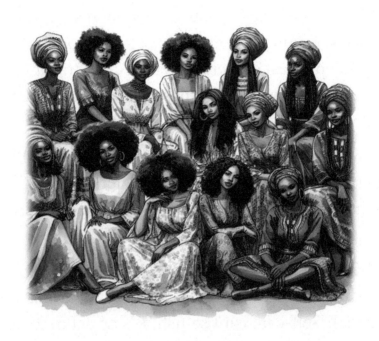

*Dedicated to all the remarkable
women out there.*

A HEARTFELT MESSAGE FROM
TIA AND TUTI

Dear Sisters,

Breast cancer awareness is important year-round, not just in October. Let's show compassion and promote regular screening and early detection throughout the year. Keep breast cancer awareness close to our hearts and take action to support those affected. Here's what we hold dear:

Awareness Matters: Breast cancer is a shared experience among mothers, daughters, friends, and neighbors. Early detection is crucial. Let's discuss breast health openly and dispel fear.

Self-Care is Self-Love: Prioritize yourself. Regular screenings, mammograms, and self-exams are essential. Self-care isn't selfish; it's an act of love.

Educate and Empower: Share facts, dispel myths, and ignite curiosity about breast health. Regular mammograms detect breast cancer early. Together, we prioritize breast health and dispel isolation.

Celebrate Survivors: Warriors wear scars as badges of courage. Each scar tells a story of bravery. Tia and Tuti believe in sharing these tales.

Spread Awareness: Educate others about early detection. Engage in events, ignite conversations, and advocate for breast health.

Breast cancer affects us all—mothers, sisters, friends. Together, we infuse hope and meaning. Tia and Tuti Tender-Heart, stand by your side, dear sisters. Let our empathy sway through the seasons: spring's renewal, summer's warmth, fall's reflection, and winter's quiet strength.

Sending warm wishes and pink ribbon hugs,

Tia and Tuti Tender-Heart

TIMELESS GENERATIONAL BONDS

In the depth of memory, three characters—Millie, Tia, and Tuti Tender-Heart—emerge. Their stories intertwine across generations, connecting hearts with hope.

Millie, a brave woman, valiantly battled breast cancer with courage. Though she is no longer with us, her legacy lives on. Her spirit continues to inspire, shaping hearts and minds through the memories and inspiration she left behind.

Tia, Millie's daughter, clung to memories like fragile threads. She held onto shared laughter, quiet conversations, and the warmth of her mother's embrace. Grief threatened to unravel those threads, leaving her adrift in a sea of loss. In those moments, Tia sought solace in her mother's courage, weaving it into her existence—a testament to the enduring power of love and hope.

Meet Tuti Tender-Heart, a cherished doll with bright eyes and a stitched smile. Beyond fabric and stuffing, she embodied hope—a silent companion for Tia. Clutched close, they embarked on a mission—a journey driven by love and guided by hope.

Tia's purpose became clear: to raise awareness about breast cancer, honor her mother's memory, and support others in their battle. She organized walks, fundraisers, and support groups with Tuti Tender-Heart silently witnessing the strength of the human spirit by her side.

Dear reader, I blend reality and fiction, drawing from personal experiences and imagination to craft these words. I weave threads of hope, delicate yet unbreakable, bridging the gap between what was and what could be. I invite you to step beyond the confines of autobiographical fiction and meet the individuals who inspired my writing—the heartbeat of these pages.

MILLIE

Mildred Hazel Walker, whom I affectionately
called "Hazel," was my older sister.

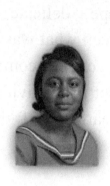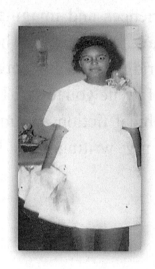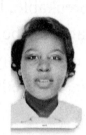

Our sisterhood and friendship remained unbreakable
from childhood to adulthood. Hazel, a born leader,
fearlessly stepped out to make a difference. Her love
for children, a cherished trait she passed on to her
daughters, remains etched in our hearts. Despite
battling breast cancer, Hazel's spirit shone brightly.
At the tender age of 39, she left this earthly realm, but
her courage continues to inspire us. Hazel embodied
strength and determination, qualities we will forever
honor and carry forward.

TIA

Cynethea Cunningham, The Author

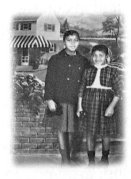 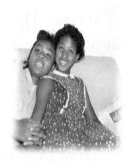 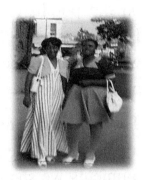

Hazel, my older sister, was always my protector. While I was more reserved, she was adventurous and outgoing. Summer trips to our grandparents' farm in North Carolina are memories I'll never forget. As city girls, it was a new and exciting experience for us. We spent our days with chickens, pigs, and horses, and woke up each morning to the sound of roosters.

Hazel quickly adapted to farm life, running through the fields with boundless energy. She taught me how to feed the chickens and even convinced me to ride a horse for the first time. I climbed up on the wooden fence to mount the horse, holding the reins with confidence while I clung on nervously behind her. We explored the vast cornfields, getting lost in the tall stalks and playing hide and seek. Our granddad was delighted, taking us on tractor rides with bales of hay that we sat on, while grandma's fried chicken and homemade biscuits with molasses were treats we eagerly looked forward to. In the evenings, we'd sit on the porch, watching the sunset and listening to Hazel's imaginative stories. Those moments, filled with laughter and family warmth, are etched in my memory forever.

Those sunny summer days of our youth are treasured memories of love, laughter, and our sisterly bond. The moments we shared—laughing, crying, arguing, and making up—remain vivid. These are memories that define our unbreakable bond.

TUTI TENDER-HEART

"Making A Difference With A Doll"

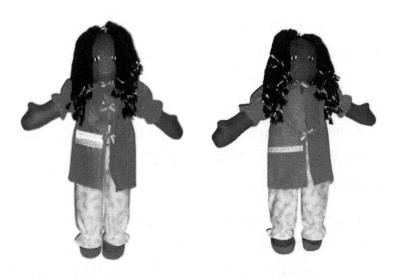

In 1987, while serving as missionaries in Liberia, West Africa, my husband Byron and I had our first encounter with breast cancer. It was unexpected and deeply personal. Our service area was about 80 miles from Monrovia, and we would visit the city once a month to shop, make phone calls at the telecommunications office, and pick up mail.

During a routine visit to the post office, I received an urgent letter from my mother: "Hazel has cancer, and the doctors have done all they can do. She's waiting for you to come home and take care of things."

Numbness, sadness, and anxiety overwhelmed me. I called my mother, who confirmed that Hazel's advanced cancer meant time was running out. Swiftly boarding a flight homeward, my heart raced—would I arrive in time?

Thankfully, I arrived in time and was grateful for those precious 11 days by her side. Then, in the early morning of September 12th, the chaplain called to inform me that "Millie," as her Palliative Care team affectionately called her, "has passed away." Though my heart was heavy with grief, I found solace in knowing she was now at peace.

Returning to Liberia to complete our mission assignment provided me with the space to grieve and process everything that had unfolded. The weight of my sister's battle with breast cancer, the urgency of her situation, and the impending loss all settled upon me during those moments. In the familiar landscape of Liberia and among the echoes of our shared memories, I grappled with the depth of my emotions. Through moments of introspection, I realized that pain, when faced with inner strength, can grow into purpose. Despite the twists and turns of life's journey, they often lead us to greater understanding and compassion.

In the years that followed, despite health challenges and the ache of my sister's absence, I lovingly crafted a doll and named her "Tuti Tender-Heart." Within her stitched seams, she held a delicate balance of emotions—both happiness and sadness. As I threaded each memory, I discovered that pain, like a gentle sculptor, molds us toward purpose. Our darkest moments transform into fertile soil for growth and compassion.

Tuti Tender-Heart, a unique cloth doll, emerged from threads of love and purpose. As a comfort doll, she weaves therapeutic solace for hearts of all ages. Holding her close, you'll find your spirits lifted and your days brightened. Her gentle smile and expression convey our shared emotions, whispering that we have the power to turn moments of sorrow into joy.

Tuti, however, wears more than just fabric; she represents a cause. Dressed in pink, with braided hair adorned with pink ribbons, she stands as a perpetual symbol: Early Detection Saves Lives. She shines a light in the darkness of breast cancer, offering hope even in difficult circumstances.

Celebrating the enduring impact
of treasured memories.

INK OF MEMORIES

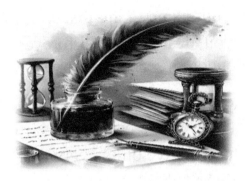

In the quiet corners of my heart,
Where memories bloom like fragile flowers,
I find you there Hazel, my sister, my friend,
A tapestry of love woven through life's hours.

Your laughter echoes on sun-kissed days,
Your courage is etched in the fabric of time,
You moved with grace through storms and haze,
A melody of strength, forever sublime.

In dreams, we walk hand in hand,
Through fields of sunflowers and endless skies,
Your spirit, a compass, forever grand,
Guiding me toward hope when sorrow tries.

So here, at the close of this written tale,
I pen your name in ink that won't fade,
For you, dear sister will forever sail,
In the boundless sea of memories, we made.

Resting now, sweet soul, in realms of endless light,
Where stars weave stories of love's embrace,
And know that you live on in every beat of my heart,
A cherished chapter, of heavenly grace.

With Love and Remembrance,

Cynethea

REFERENCES

1. American Cancer Society. "Breast Cancer Facts & Figures 2019-2020." Accessed from. https://www.cancer.org/research/cancer-facts-statistics/breast-cancer-facts-figures.html. Pg. 45.

2. DeSantis, C.E., et al. (2019). "Breast cancer statistics, 2019." CA: A Cancer Journal for Clinicians, 69(6), 438-451. Pg. 45.

3. https://www.cancer.org/research/acs-research-news/facts-and-figures-african-american-black-people-2022-2024/html. Pg. 45.

ACKNOWLEDGMENTS

I want to express my heartfelt gratitude to everyone who has supported me on my writing journey.

Jackie Stanley, your support was a lifeline. Thank you for your prayers and encouragement over the years. Your open heart and welcoming home provided us with much-needed respite. It was within those walls that Tuti Tender-Heart found her voice, a genuine reflection of your kindness.

Chase, your input during Tuti's creation has been incredibly helpful! Your writing expertise and encouragement as my nephew have been a driving force that inspired me to keep pushing forward.

Katrinka, your encouragement, guidance, and expertise have been invaluable to me. Your support has made a significant difference throughout my journey, and I am deeply grateful.

Deborah, Quincey, Katrinka, Alisa, Micah, and Chamesia, thank you for being a part of the initial Tuti Tender-Heart project. Your enthusiasm and heartfelt contributions shaped its very essence. We were dreamers back then, and now in 2024, the time has arrived!

Bishop Luther Baker, I want to express my deep gratitude for your commitment to sharing spiritual wisdom and uplifting the body of Christ. Your words of inspiration and transformative impact have enriched my journey and continue to inspire me. Thank you for your profound influence.

To all the readers who have joined me on this journey, whether you're holding a physical copy of this book or scrolling through its digital pages, I want to express my sincere gratitude. Your curiosity, empathy, and open hearts have given life to these words. You have transformed mere ink and paper into a shared experience, and for that, I am profoundly thankful.

To all the quiet supporters, late-night readers, and borrowed book enthusiasts—I want you to know that I see you. You are the unsung heroes of this story. Your presence, even in anonymity, has created connections across time and space. Thank you and may these words resonate with you wherever you are.

Dedicated to Millie, who faced breast cancer with grace and courage, this book honors your enduring legacy. Tuti, our tender-hearted doll, symbolizes hope, healing, and the unbreakable bond between a mother and her child.

To all the resilient Millies facing breast cancer, your courage and strength shine brightly in difficult times. In the quiet moments of struggle, you embody hope and healing. Your spirit teaches us that strength isn't always loud; sometimes, it's a gentle whisper echoing through our hearts.

May your journey be filled with compassion, understanding, and support. As we weave your stories into the fabric of Tuti Tender-Heart, know that we see, cherish, and celebrate you. Your graceful legacy inspires us all.

May this book be a vessel of compassion, shelter for weary souls, and a testament to the power of storytelling. Together, we honor the past, embrace the present, and step boldly into the future.

A MESSAGE OF HOPE AND SUPPORT

Dear Reader,

As the author of "Tuti Tender-Heart And The Journey Of Hope," I want to take a moment to speak directly to those who are fighting breast cancer and to the survivors who have bravely faced this journey. Your strength, determination, and courage are truly inspiring.

Having witnessed the journey of loved ones through breast cancer, I understand the challenges and triumphs that come with it. There is a dear friend who comes to mind, someone who always managed to inspire others and bring light into their lives. Despite the grueling treatments, she showed that hope and love can prevail. This book is devoted to you, and I hope it brings comfort and encouragement.

To those who wish to support cancer fighters and survivors, here are some thoughtful ways to offer encouragement:

Personal Messages: Simple, heartfelt messages can uplift spirits. Phrases like "You're stronger than you know" or "One day at a time, you've got this" can be very powerful.

Inspirational Quotes: Share quotes that inspire hope and strength. For example, "Cancer cannot cripple love, it cannot shatter hope, it cannot conquer the spirit."

Care Packages: Send a care package with comforting items like a cozy blanket, books, or snacks.

Meals and Errands: Offer to bring meals or help with errands. This can ease their daily burdens and show that you care.

Listen Actively: Sometimes, just being there to listen can be incredibly comforting. Let them share their feelings without judgment.

Support Groups: Encourage them to join support groups where they can connect with others who understand their experiences.

Letters and Cards: Write letters or send cards regularly to remind them they are in your thoughts.

Arts and Music: Share uplifting art or music that can provide a mental escape and boost their mood.

Financial Support: If possible, offer financial assistance for medical bills or daily expenses.

Volunteer: Get involved with organizations that support cancer patients and survivors.

Incorporating these gestures into your interactions can provide much-needed comfort and strength for those fighting breast cancer. Together, we can make a meaningful impact on their journey. Every act of kindness, no matter how small, contributes to a larger network of support and love. Let's stand unified, offering hope and compassion, and remind those affected by breast cancer that they are never alone. Together, we can create a brighter, more hopeful future for all.

With all my heart,

Cynethea

ABOUT THE AUTHOR

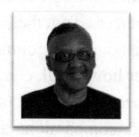

Cynethea Cunningham is a versatile artist—Artisan, Author, and Poet. Her creativity shines through various mediums. As a self-taught seamstress, crocheter, greeting card designer, and doll-maker, she crafts magic with her hands. However, her true passion is writing. Through prose and poetry, she paints vivid landscapes of ideas and imagination. Her poems, like delicate tapestries, weave tales that resonate with the soul.

Cynethea's dedication to breast cancer advocacy is truly inspiring. Her Tuti Tender-Heart Breast Cancer Awareness doll received Copyright Certification in 2008 and a Trademark in 2010. In 2011, Cynethea was honored with a Proclamation Certificate from the Prince George's County Council, recognizing her tireless efforts to educate the public about breast cancer awareness.

Cynethea and Ward, residents of Rockville, MD, have shared a beautiful love story that has flourished through 48 years of marriage, marked by 45 years of devoted service in Christian ministry. They have been blessed with two sons: Andre, who resides in the Maryland area, and their youngest son, Brandon, who now rests with the Lord.

ALSO BY CYNETHEA CUNNINGHAM

"Growing in Christ: Steps to a Firm Foundation" is a Bible study workbook focused on key aspects of the Christian faith like Salvation, Baptism, and Communion. It provides clear guidance to children, helping them understand these important elements as they grow in their relationship with Jesus. This workbook is a valuable resource for parents, Sunday School teachers and children's ministry leaders to support spiritual growth.

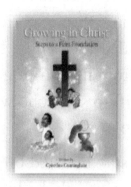 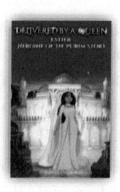

"Delivered By A Queen: Esther Heroine of the Purim Story" is a captivating book about the biblical story of Purim. It highlights Queen Esther's bravery as she risked her life to save her people. Although God's name isn't mentioned, His presence is felt throughout the story, turning a day of potential destruction into a celebration. The book, based on the ten chapters of Esther, is written as an engaging and educational poem with added insights.

You can find them on Amazon. Happy reading!

WILL YOU DO ME A FAVOR?

If you enjoyed reading "Tuti Tender-Heart And The Journey of Hope" as much as I enjoyed writing it, I would deeply appreciate it if you could take a moment to leave a review on Amazon. Reviews play a crucial role in helping others discover titles they may also enjoy.

Also, if this book has touched your heart and it has blessed you, consider sharing that experience with others. You can recommend it to friends, family, or anyone who might benefit from its uplifting message. Even sending a copy as a gift to someone would be a wonderful way to spread the joy.

Follow me on Amazon to stay updated on my latest releases and special offers. Just click the 'Follow' button on my Amazon Author Page.

Thank you sincerely for your support.

Made in the USA
Columbia, SC
09 November 2024

45604817R00085